75 Questions & Answers About Lymphoma

Second Edition

Updated Edition

Peter Holman, MD
Moores Cancer Center
University of California, San Diego

Jodi Garrett, RN
Moores Cancer Center
University of California, San Diego

JONES & BARTLETT
LEARNING

World Headquarters
Jones & Bartlett Learning
5 Wall Street
Burlington, MA 01803
info@jblearning.com
www.jblearning.com

Jones & Bartlett Learning books and products are available through most bookstores and online booksellers. To contact Jones & Bartlett Learning directly, call 800-832-0034, fax 978-443-8000, or visit our website, www.jblearning.com.

Substantial discounts on bulk quantities of Jones & Bartlett Learning publications are available to corporations, professional associations, and other qualified organizations. For details and specific discount information, contact the special sales department at Jones & Bartlett Learning via the above contact information or send an email to specialsale@jblearning.com.

The authors, editor, and publisher have made every effort to provide accurate information. However, they are not responsible for errors, omissions, or for any outcomes related to the use of the contents of this book and take no responsibility for the use of the products and procedures described. Treatments and side effects described in this book may not be applicable to all people; likewise, some people may require a dose or experience a side effect that is not described herein. Drugs and medical devices are discussed that may have limited availability controlled by the Food and Drug Administration (FDA) for use only in a research study or clinical trial. Research, clinical practice, and government regulations often change the accepted standard in this field. When consideration is being given to use of any drug in the clinical setting, the healthcare provider or reader is responsible for determining FDA status of the drug, reading the package insert, and reviewing prescribing information for the most up-to-date recommendations on dose, precautions, and contraindications, and determining the appropriate usage for the product. This is especially important in the case of drugs that are new or seldom used.

Production Credits
Executive Publisher: Christopher Davis
Managing Editor, Custom Projects: Kathy Richardson
Associate Production Editor: Tina Chen
Marketing Manager: Rebecca Rockel
Manufacturing and Inventory Control Supervisor: Amy Bacus
Composition: Abella Publishing Services
Cover Design: Carolyn Downer
Cover Images: Clockwise, from top left: © Sparkling Moments Photography/ShutterStock, Inc.; © AbleStock; © lucwa/ShutterStock, Inc.
Printing and Binding: Malloy, Inc.
Cover Printing: Malloy, Inc.

6048

Printed in the United States of America
15 14 13 12 11 10 9 8 7 6 5 4 3 2 1

Contents

Introduction

According to the American Cancer Society, approximately 74,490 new cases of lymphoma will be diagnosed in the United States in 2009. Of these, approximately 65,980 cases will be non-Hodgkin's lymphoma, and the remaining cases (8,510) will be Hodgkin's disease. Since the early 1970s, for unclear reasons, the incidence of lymphoma has doubled and continues to rise.

The term "lymphoma" actually describes many different but related diseases. Although there is overlap, the different lymphomas tend to affect people in different ways. There are even some types of lymphoma that may not always require treatment; for most lymphomas, however, there are a number of treatment choices that can be made in any particular situation. It is therefore a major challenge for individuals receiving such a diagnosis to obtain the relevant information necessary to be an active participant in their care. The Internet is a very useful source of information, but it also contains much disinformation that can be more damaging and frightening than helpful.

In this book, written for patients and their caregivers, we (a physician and a nurse) have attempted to provide an understanding of lymphoma that will assist you in understanding this disease and coping with the daily pressures of the fight against lymphoma. In addition, the Appendix includes links to sites with additional information about lymphoma-related clinical research and clinical trials. We hope you find it useful.

Peter Holman, MD
Jodi Garrett, RN

PART ONE

The Basics: Understanding the Immune and Circulatory Systems

What is the immune system?

How do the components of the immune system function?

What is bone marrow?

More . . .

1. What is the immune system?

All types of **lymphoma** arise from cells that are part of the normal **immune system**. Understanding the immune system is therefore important to understanding lymphoma. Your immune system is what protects you from illnesses by recognizing and eliminating dangerous foreign (abnormal) substances. This system is your main defense against all infections (illness arising from invasion from an outside organism, such as **bacteria** or **viruses**) and also plays an important role in how your body responds to many diseases, including lymphoma and other cancers. Individuals in whom the immune system is not functioning properly have an increased risk of certain cancers (including lymphoma), infections, and autoimmune disorders, which are illnesses characterized by organ damage as a result of self-recognition by cells of the immune system.

The immune system consists of a variety of important components, including a meshwork-like circulation system of **lymphatic channels** throughout the body that connect the **lymph nodes** or **lymph glands**, the **tonsils**, the **spleen**, and the **thymus** (Figure 1) and is in series with the blood circulation and also the **bone marrow**. The spleen is an organ that is normally the size of your fist and can become enlarged when affected by lymphoma. It essentially functions like a very large lymph node and is located in the upper left abdomen, beside the stomach. The thymus is another lymphoid organ that is located behind the breastbone (sternum) in children and young adults; it becomes inactive in older adults. The circulating **lymph fluid** contains large numbers of **lymphocytes**—white blood cells that fight disease. The lymphocytes are the "foot

Lymphoma
cancer of the lymphocytes.

Immune system
the complex system by which the body protects itself from harmful outside invaders.

Bacteria
one class of infectious agents.

Viruses
tiny infectious agents that require other cells for their growth and survival.

Lymphatic channels
the tiny vessels that connect the lymph glands.

Lymph nodes
another term for lymph glands.

Lymph glands
the large collections of lymphocytes present at intervals throughout the lymph system. They can get big and painful in response to an infection.

Tonsils
large lymph nodes present in the back of the throat.

Spleen
the large lymph node–like organ under the lower left ribs.

soldiers" of the immune system, directly responsible for destroying invading organisms or abnormal cells.

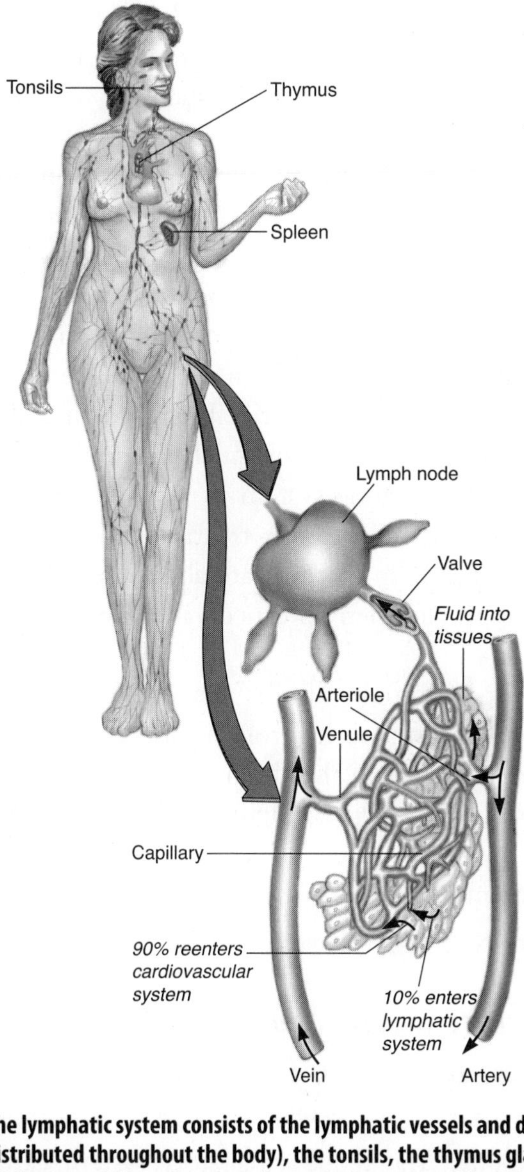

Figure 1 The lymphatic system consists of the lymphatic vessels and ducts, lymph nodes (which are distributed throughout the body), the tonsils, the thymus gland, and the spleen. The enlarged diagram of a lymph node and vessels shows the path of the excess fluid that leaves the arteriole end of a capillary bed, enters the adjacent tissue spaces, and is absorbed by lymphatic capillaries. Reprinted from Alters: *Biology: Understanding Life*, Fourth Ed. Copyright © 2000 Jones and Bartlett Publishers, LLC.

Thymus
an organ behind the breastbone that is important for the development of an immune response, especially in children.

Bone marrow
soft substance inside many bones in the body where the blood cells are produced.

Lymph fluid
the fluid that carries lymphocytes around the body.

Lymphocytes
the main type of cell that makes up the immune system and is the abnormal cell in lymphoma.

B cell
a type of lymphocyte.

T cell
one of the major types of lymphocytes.

Tissues
a collection of cells of a similar type with a similar function.

Autoimmune disease
an illness in which a person's own immune system can recognize parts of its own body as foreign.

The two main types of lymphocytes (**B cells** and **T cells**) act together with other immune cells to mount an attack in response to foreign invaders such as infections. The manner in which disease cells are recognized is essential in the body's success or failure in fending off an illness. For example, under certain circumstances, lymphocytes mistake an individual's own body **tissues** for foreign substances. In such cases, this error results in an immune attack on normal tissues; such attacks are called an **autoimmune disease** and include illnesses such as **rheumatoid arthritis** and **systemic lupus erythematosus**. It is important to note that in most cancers, including lymphoma, the immune system fails in the opposite way—it does not recognize the cancer cells as foreign and therefore allows the cancer to grow unchecked. Clearly, the ability of the immune system to respond appropriately is one key factor in cancer treatment, and failure of the immune system to eradicate abnormal cells may result in the development of cancers including lymphoma.

The body initially "trains" its own T cells to distinguish foreign proteins from normal body proteins. This training occurs in the thymus during childhood, when the thymus is still an active organ; after adolescence, the thymus shrinks (or involutes) and has little or no function in adults.

2. How do the components of the immune system function?

Two circulatory systems transport immune cells around the body. The blood circulatory system carries blood from the heart to the lungs, where **red blood cells** receive oxygen, and then onward via the **arteries** throughout the body where oxygen and nutrients are delivered to tissues, allowing normal metabolism to occur. At the same time, carbon dioxide, waste, and toxic matter are transported to the lungs, liver, or kidneys for elimination from the body. In addition to this function of supplying oxygen and removing waste substances, the blood also carries the disease- and injury-fighting white blood cells, which include the lymphocytes and a number of other cells (described in Questions 4 and 5), as well as many other types of protein, including those that are important for blood clotting.

The lesser known circulatory system is the lymphatic circulatory system, which works alongside the blood circulatory system in fighting disease. The lymphatic circulation transports the lymph fluid—rich in lymphocytes around the body—in lymph channels in much the same way as blood is transported via arteries and **veins**. Lymphocytes are produced in the bone marrow (see Question 3), after which they travel through both the bloodstream and lymphatic channels to the lymph nodes and/or the thymus (in children and adolescents) and then back into the bloodstream. The lymphatic channels that compose the lymphatic circulatory system consist of tiny, thin, leaky vessels that carry lymph fluid back toward the heart. They usually run alongside the veins, which likewise carry blood back to the heart from various parts of the body.

At frequent intervals along the lymphatic channels, large clusters of lymphocytes occur. These are the lymph nodes or glands in which lymphocytes often first encounter a foreign protein or **antigen**. When a lymphocyte recognizes a protein as foreign, it sends out signals to other lymphocytes, recruiting help in mounting an immune response directed at ridding the

Rheumatoid arthritis
an autoimmune disorder associated with destruction and deformity of joints.

Systemic lupus erythematosus
a disease in which the immune system attacks the body.

Red blood cells
the most common type of blood cells that carry oxygen around the body.

Arteries
the vessels that carry blood containing oxygen to the organs and tissues of the body.

Veins
blood vessels that return blood to the heart.

Antigen
any substance that can induce an immune response. This could be an infection or a cancer cell.

body of the foreign protein. Lymphocytes and other inflammatory cells accumulate in the region, and when activated through their encounter with the foreign substance, they secrete chemical messengers that orchestrate the appropriate immune response. An example of this is the development of red, swollen tonsils (which are large lymphatic organs in the throat) during an infection or a cold. Similarly, lymph nodes in other sites can become enlarged and painful during a serious infection. This accumulation reflects the immune system's attempt to control and eliminate the infection. Lymph nodes are located throughout the body, but, when enlarged, they are most easily felt in the neck, armpits, and groin. Collections of nodes also occur in the chest, between the lungs, and in the abdomen, where they are found alongside the **aorta** and the **inferior vena cava**, the major blood vessels, which carry blood away from and back to the heart.

Aorta

the main blood vessel (artery) that carries blood from the heart to the smaller arteries, delivering blood to all parts of the body.

Inferior vena cava

the large vein that carries blood back toward the heart.

The spleen is a specialized organ within the immune system and functions in many respects as a very large lymph node. The spleen is essentially a very large collection of lymphocytes and is another site where lymphocytes can come into contact with foreign proteins. Certain infections, including **infectious mononucleosis** (commonly called glandular fever) and **malaria**, can result in an enlarged spleen. When this occurs, your physician may feel the spleen (when it is a normal size, it cannot be felt) when examining your abdomen. Under certain circumstances, the spleen needs to be surgically removed. If this is necessary, especially in children, antibiotics may be prescribed to prevent certain types of infection. Although you can live a normal life without a spleen, it is an important part of the immune system, providing significant protection

Infectious mononucleosis

a viral infection caused by the Epstein-Barr virus. Also called glandular fever.

Malaria

an infection caused by a parasite and transmitted by mosquitoes.

against some types of infection; thus, patients without a spleen should seek medical attention quickly in the event of an infection.

You can think of these components as a defensive army that is fighting a continuing battle against would-be invaders. The lymphocyte "ground troops" are armed within the bone marrow (during childhood, they are also sent out for "training" in the thymus). Then they patrol the body via the lymphatic system and battle invaders in the nodes and, during cases of very serious invasion, in the tonsils and spleen as well.

3. What is bone marrow?

The bone marrow is the soft substance that is present inside many of the bones in your body. It is where all blood cells are produced from the blood-forming **stem cells**, responsible for the production of red blood cells, white blood cells, and **platelets**. All of these cells go though a number of different stages of maturation within the bone marrow before mature cells are released into the bloodstream. If the bloodstream becomes deficient in any type of cell, such as a low red blood cell count in a patient with **anemia**, the bone marrow may attempt to replace the missing red blood cells by increasing production. Bone marrow is present in the skull, backbone (vertebrae), ribs, hips, and pelvic bones and at the top ends of the **humerus** (upper arm bone) and **femur** (thigh bone). Normally, fat cells take up approximately half the bone marrow space; the other half consists of the blood-forming cells. The bone marrow can be involved in many types of lymphoma, explaining the need for bone marrow examinations.

Stem cells

the cells that can produce red blood cells, white blood cells, and platelets.

Platelets

the tiny blood cells that are produced in the bone marrow and are important for blood clotting.

Anemia

a low hemoglobin level.

Humerus

the major bone connecting the shoulder to the elbow.

Femur

the thigh bone.

4. *What are lymphocytes?*

Lymphocytes are one type of white blood cell (other white blood cells are described in Question 5; see Figure 2). Although they fight disease, lymphocytes are the "foot soldiers" of the immune system, and it is specifically these cells that lymphoma affects (Question 1). The two main types of lymphocytes, B and T cells, have different roles in working to eliminate foreign proteins (antigens) from the body, but they work together to achieve the same result of preventing and eliminating illnesses.

B lymphocytes (or B cells) are named for where they come from in chicken embryos—an organ called the "bursa of Fabricious," although humans have no such organ. Both B and T lymphocytes are produced in our bone marrow. T lymphocytes (or T cells) are so called because of the important role that the thymus plays in their development.

From the bone marrow, T cells circulate throughout the body using both blood vessels and lymphatic channels. T and B cells look identical when blood is examined under a microscope, but the types of molecules or protein substances on their surface can help to distinguish them. Specialized laboratory equipment found in most hospitals or clinical laboratories can be used to distinguish the different types of lymphocytes on the basis of these proteins. It is the growth and accumulation of large numbers of abnormal lymphocytes that result in the lymph node enlargement that occurs in lymphoma.

Natural Killer Cells

Natural killer (NK) cells are a type of lymphocyte and account for most of the large granular lymphocytes present in the blood. Abnormalities result in a number of types of lymphoma or leukemia. These types of lymphoma are rare. NK cells play an important role in the function of the immune system. If an individual is born without NK cells, death results from severe infection.

5. What are the other types of blood cells?

In addition to lymphocytes, the bone marrow produces many other types of blood cells (Figure 2) that are the offspring of a very important bone marrow cell called the **hematopoietic stem cell**, which can produce all of the blood cells ("hematopoietic" is derived from the Greek words *haimatos*, which means blood, and *poiein*, which means to make). Embryonic stem cells, the subject of much ongoing scientific, ethical, and political discussion, differ from these cells, as they can give rise to cells of many more different tissues than the hematopoietic stem cell. Thus, when stem cells are discussed in this context, we mean strictly the hematopoietic stem cells that give rise to blood cells.

Hematopoietic stem cell
the most immature cell that develops into red blood cells, white blood cells, and platelets.

The main groups of blood cells are red cells, white cells, and platelets. As mentioned previously, the B and T lymphocytes are only two of a number of different types of **white blood cells**.

White blood cells
blood cells that are most important for fighting infection.

White Blood Cells

All of the white blood cells are produced in the bone marrow. From there, they make their way into the bloodstream, where they circulate for varying lengths of time before moving into the tissues of the body. They can carry out their functions in the bloodstream or various tissues.

		BLOOD CELL TYPE	DESCRIPTION	FUNCTION	LIFE SPAN
RED BLOOD CELLS		Erythrocyte 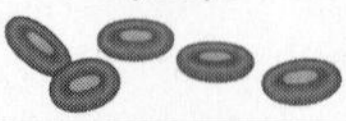	Flat disk with a central depression, no nucleus, contain hemoglobin.	Transport oxygen (O_2) and carbon dioxide (CO_2).	About 120 days.
WHITE BLOOD CELLS (LEUKOCYTES)	Granulocytes	Neutrophil 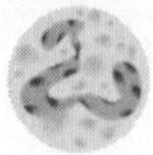	Spherical; with many-lobed nucleus, no hemoglobin, pink-purple **cytoplasmic granules**.	Cellular defense-phagocytosis of small microorganisms.	Hours to 3 days.
	Granulocytes	Eosinophil 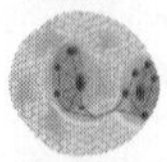	Spherical; two-lobed nucleus, no hemoglobin, orange-red staining **cytoplasmic granules**.	Cellular defense—phagocytosis of large microorganisms such as parasitic worms, releases anti-inflammatory substances in allergic reactions.	8 to 12 days.
	Granulocytes	Basophil 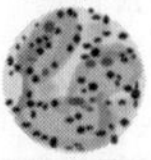	Spherical; generally two-lobed nucleus, no hemoglobin large purple staining **cytoplasmic granules**.	Inflammatory response–contain granules that rupture and release chemicals enhancing inflammatory response.	Hours to 3 days.
	Agranulocytes	Monocyte 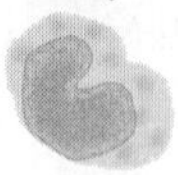	Spherical; **single nucleus** shaped like kidney bean, no cytoplasmic granules, cytoplasm often blue in color.	Converted to macrophages, which are large cells that entrap microorganisms and other foreign matter.	Days to months.
	Agranulocytes	B lymphocyte 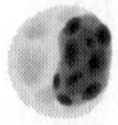	Spherical; round **singular nucleus**, no cytoplasmic granules.	Immune system response and regulation, antibody production sometimes causes allergic response.	Days to years.
	Agranulocytes	T lymphocyte 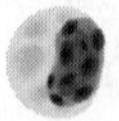	Spherical; round **singular nucleus**, no cytoplasmic granules.	Immune system response and regulation; cellular immune response.	Days to years.
PLATELETS		Platelets 	Irregularly shaped fragments, very small pink staining granules.	Control blood clotting or coagulation.	7 to 10 days.

Figure 2 Types of blood cells. Reprinted from Alters: *Biology: Understanding Life*, Fourth Ed. Copyright © 2000 Jones and Bartlett Publishers, LLC.

Neutrophil

the main white blood cell important for fighting infection.

Nucleus

the central part of the cell that contains the genetic information.

Cytoplasm

the part of a cell that surrounds the central nucleus.

Neutrophils, a particularly important cell in defense against bacterial infections, are the most common type of white blood cell. Lymphocytes are the second most frequent white blood cell. Neutrophils are easily identified under a microscope with a **nucleus** that is divided up into three or four lobes. The **cytoplasm** (the part of the cell that surrounds the nucleus) of the neutrophils contains **granules**, which in turn contain chemicals (**enzymes**) that are important for killing bacteria. When someone has a bacterial infection, the number of white cells in the blood normally increases, mostly because of an increase in neutrophils.

Chemotherapy, which is a name for medications used to treat disease—cancer, in this case—can be used to kill the cancer cells, but it can also prevent the bone marrow's production of neutrophils. In general, cells that turn over rapidly (having a higher proliferation rate) are more sensitive to the effects of chemotherapy. Neutrophils have a high proliferation, and, thus, people receiving chemotherapy have periods when they are at an increased risk of bacterial infection. For this reason, many patients on chemotherapy also receive **growth factors**, which increase the neutrophil count, and/or antibiotics, in an attempt to prevent infections.

Granules
small particles containing enzymes.

Enzymes
chemical messengers within the body.

Chemotherapy
drugs used to treat a disease; the different types of drugs used to treat cancer.

Growth factors
chemicals that can be injected to stimulate the production of blood cells.

Other white blood cells include **monocytes**, **eosinophils**, and **basophils**. The monocytes are also important in preventing and controlling bacterial infections. Eosinophils are important in responding to parasites and have a role in allergic reactions. The white blood cell count is usually normal in people when they are diagnosed with lymphoma, but some types of lymphoma can first be identified by the finding of an elevated white blood cell count. It is important to know which types of white blood cells are present in the blood, as even when the white blood cell count is normal, lymphoma cells can be found circulating in the blood. When tested in a clinical laboratory, the white blood cell count is reported as an absolute number, and a differential count is usually given, identifying the relative percentage of neutrophils, lymphocytes, eosinophils, and basophils. The absolute number of the different white blood cells can then be calculated.

Monocytes
a type of white blood cell.

Eosinophils
a type of white blood cell.

Basophils
a type of white blood cell.

Red Blood Cells

Red blood cells, the most common type of blood cells, do not have a nucleus but contain a red pigment called **hemoglobin**, which is essential to life

Hemoglobin
a protein present in red blood cells that carries oxygen.

because it allows oxygen to be carried around the body. A low hemoglobin level indicates anemia and is easily determined by performing a **complete blood count** (CBC). The most common reasons for people with lymphoma to develop anemia are the presence of lymphoma in the bone marrow or the effects of chemotherapy on the bone marrow.

Complete blood count
a blood test looking at the red blood cell count, the hemoglobin, the white blood cell count, and the platelet count.

Platelets

Platelets are another identifiable component of blood. They are fragments produced in the bone marrow from very large cells called **megakaryocytes**. Platelets are very important in preventing and healing bleeding and bruising. Lymphoma involving the bone marrow or chemotherapy can affect the megakaryocytic production of platelets. Rarely, low platelet counts can result from the production of autoantibodies that bind to platelets. These antibody-coated platelets then get removed from the circulation by the spleen. Signs of a low platelet count include easy or spontaneous bruising, nose bleeding (epistaxis), or menstrual periods that are heavier than normal (menorrhagia). Platelet transfusions may be warranted to reduce the risk of bleeding or to stop bleeding under certain circumstances.

Megakaryocytes
the bone marrow cells that produce platelets.

The platelet count can also sometimes be high in patients with lymphoma or other cancers, as the body may react to the presence of cancer, infection, or some types of inflammation by releasing chemicals or **cytokines** that stimulate megakaryocytes to make more platelets. With treatment, the platelet count will generally return to normal.

Cytokines
chemicals produced by T lymphocytes to generate an immune response.

6. *How does the immune system fight infection?*

The immune system has two main overlapping strategies to defend against foreign proteins. One approach uses the **humoral immune response**, and the foot soldiers for this mode of attack are the B cells. The other approach is the **cellular immune response**, which employs predominantly T cells. The two strategies generally act in concert to eliminate a foreign substance.

The humoral immune response uses **antibodies** to eliminate foreign protein. Antibodies are Y-shaped proteins. Each arm can attach to the foreign protein in much the same way as a key fits in a lock. The arms of the Y bind to the foreign protein, and the leg attaches to another type of immune cell called a **phagocyte**, which then removes the foreign protein coated with antibody from the circulation. **Monoclonal antibodies** used in the treatment of lymphoma and other cancers are designed to interact with targets on the surface of lymphoma cells or other cancer cells, bringing them together with normal immune system cells in an attempt to kill the cancer cells.

When specific B cells interact with and recognize a substance as foreign, they receive signals to develop into antibody-secreting cells. These cells are called **plasma cells**, which are found mostly in the spleen but are also common in the bone marrow. Normally, there is one pool of B cells for each different foreign protein that anybody might encounter over the course of a lifetime. When exposed to that foreign protein, the specific pool of B cells that can react to that foreign protein is stimulated to develop into plasma cells. The

Humoral immune response

an immune response that uses antibodies rather than cells to destroy an antigen (foreign protein).

Cellular immune response

the part of the immune response that uses lymphocytes to directly remove antigens. In contrast, the humoral immune response uses antibodies to remove antigens.

Antibodies

specialized proteins of the immune system that help fight infections. They can also be created to recognize proteins on cancer cells, as in some types of lymphoma treatments.

Phagocyte

a cell that scavenges other cells.

Monoclonal antibodies

antibodies that bind to a specific target on the surface of lymphoma or other cancer cells.

Plasma cells

the most mature type of B cell. They produce immunoglobulins.

resulting population of plasma cells produces a specific antibody that is capable of attaching itself to the foreign protein on the cell surface. The attachment of the antibody to the foreign protein marks that cell for removal from the circulation.

Some of the B cells that recognize a foreign substance do not become plasma cells but instead act to recruit T cells to help fight the foreign invader. The type of immune response that results from T cell involvement is called the cellular immune response, which does not use antibodies; instead, T cells, when activated by an encounter with the foreign protein, create chemicals called **lymphokines** that in turn activate an entire host of immune cells, including phagocytes, with the end result of eliminating the infection. Lymphokines and similar substances called cytokines are responsible for many of the symptoms, such as fever and aches, that occur during viral infections such as the flu.

Lymphokines

chemicals that are produced by lymphocytes and help in coordinating the immune response.

7. How is the immune system important in lymphoma?

The immune system is designed to recognize foreign proteins, and the way it does this is most evident in the responses seen with infection; however, the immune system also plays a role in surveying the body for abnormal cells that, if not removed, can become cancers. All cancers start out as an abnormality that occurs in a single cell. This abnormal cell develops a feature that somehow allows it to survive better than its normal counterparts—that is, it develops a survival advantage. In order to recognize an abnormal cell as foreign, the cells of the immune system need to recognize a protein on the surface of the cell as abnormal. In lymphoma and many other cancers, the proteins on the surface of the lymphoma cell appear normal, explaining why the immune response against the cancer is weak or absent.

All lymphomas arise from abnormalities in cells of the immune system, specifically the lymphocytes. It is widely thought that many tissues develop small numbers of abnormal cells that have the potential to develop into cancers, but the immune system's recognition of these cells results in their safe removal. Therefore, a failure of the immune system to recognize the abnormal cells before they become a cancer is one mechanism whereby cancers, including lymphoma, can occur.

In some types of lymphoma, characterized by slow growth and sometimes not requiring treatment for varying periods of time, the lymph node enlargement can wax and wane. This is felt to reflect the immune system's attempt to control the lymphoma. This observation suggests that ways to enhance the immune system may allow for improved control of these types of lymphoma and possibly even a cure.

The treatment of lymphoma itself can have a significant impact on the immune system. The presence of lymphoma can impair the ability of the immune system to respond to infection, and this can be improved with treatment by controlling the lymphoma; however, the treatment of the lymphoma itself can further impair the functioning of the immune system.

PART TWO

Diagnosis and Classification of Lymphoma

What is lymphoma?

What is the difference between Hodgkin's disease and non-Hodgkin's lymphoma?

What are the symptoms of lymphoma?

More . . .

8. *What is lymphoma?*

Lymphoma is cancer of the lymphatic system, specifically the lymphocytes, in which an abnormality occurs in one lymphocyte that provides the cell with a growth advantage, allowing the cell to divide and grow abnormally. Like all cancer cells, the abnormal lymphocyte does not obey the signals that control normal cell behavior. This allows more of the abnormal cells to grow, eventually developing into a large collection of the abnormal lymphocytes, which, when big enough to be detected by a physical examination or an X-ray, is called a tumor or mass. A **biopsy** can then be done that allows the lymphoma to be diagnosed.

Lymphoma
cancer of the lymphatic system, specifically the lymphocytes, in which an abnormality occurs in one lymphocyte that provides the cell with a growth advantage, allowing the cell to divide and grow abnormally.

Biopsy
the removal of tissue or a fluid sample for microscopic examination.

Most commonly, the abnormal growth of lymphocytes occurs in the lymph nodes, which then become enlarged. Abnormal lymphocytes can also collect in the bone marrow, the blood, the spleen, or other sites such as the gut, lungs, or brain. It is not uncommon for the skin to be involved.

Lymphoma is actually a very broad term that applies to many different disorders that all have many features in common (the features described here). They all arise from an abnormality occurring in a lymphocyte. There are different types of lymphocytes, and abnormalities can occur at many different stages along the normal developmental pathway. As a result, there are many different types of lymphoma that can develop, making the classification of lymphomas very complicated.

Hodgkin's disease
a type of lymphoma.

Non-Hodgkin's lymphoma
the most common type of lymphoma.

Pathologist
a physician who makes the diagnosis of lymphoma and other cancers from evaluating biopsies and other surgical specimens under the microscope.

The two main types of lymphoma are **Hodgkin's disease** and **non-Hodgkin's lymphoma**. Hodgkin's disease is named after Thomas Hodgkin, an English **pathologist** who originally described the disease in 1832.

9. What is the difference between Hodgkin's disease and non-Hodgkin's lymphoma?

Hodgkin's disease, also called Hodgkin's lymphoma, is a cancer of the lymphatic system that arises from a B lymphocyte. Non-Hodgkin's lymphomas arise most commonly from B lymphocytes, but also from T lymphocytes. There are two broad categories of Hodgkin's disease (Table 1). The first is classic Hodgkin's disease. The second, less common type is nodular lymphocyte predominant Hodgkin's disease. The distinction between these categories and between non-Hodgkin's lymphoma is made by pathological evaluation of lymph nodes. Hodgkin's disease most commonly affects people in their late teens or early 20s and people in their 50s. Non-Hodgkin's lymphomas generally increase in incidence with age. There are many different types of non-Hodgkin's lymphoma, which are discussed later.

Table 1 The different types of Hodgkin's disease

Type	Prevalence
Nodular sclerosing	Most common (75%)
Lymphocyte predominant	
Mixed cellularity	
Lymphocyte depleted	Least common (less than 5%)

10. What are the symptoms of lymphoma?

The most common presenting symptom of lymphoma is the finding of enlarged or swollen lymph nodes

Lymphadenopathy

enlarged lymph nodes.

(called **lymphadenopathy**). This most commonly is found initially in the neck, armpit, or groin, as these are areas where lymph nodes can be felt (Table 2). Enlarged lymph nodes are usually painless but more likely to be tender if they have grown very fast. The most common cause of an enlarged lymph node is an infection. Most frequently, enlarged lymph nodes within the chest or abdomen do not cause any symptoms at all.

As the lymphatic system branches all throughout the body, these swellings may occur anywhere, even in places where you or your doctor cannot feel them due to their being inaccessible. Lymph node enlargement can result in pressure effects on nearby structures. Lymph node enlargement in the groin or the axilla can result in swelling of the leg or arm on the same side. If the lymph node swelling develops in your stomach area or intestinal tract, you may have abdominal pain and/or bloating or a feeling of getting full faster than normal. When the lymph nodes in the chest become involved, cough, shortness of breath, or chest pain may develop. Sometimes, if the lymph nodes in the center of the chest get big very fast, they can cause **superior vena cava syndrome**, which is a result of pressure that the lymph nodes put on veins, resulting in slowing

Superior vena cava syndrome

a condition in which the blood flow back to the heart is decreased due to obstruction, usually by very big lymph nodes.

Table 2 The symptoms of lymphoma

Lymphoma symptoms are not specific. Not all people with lymphoma will experience all symptoms, and some will have symptoms not listed here. Common symptoms include:

- Fatigue
- Painless swelling of lymph glands
- Fevers
- Night sweats
- Weight loss

of the blood flow returning from your arms and head back to your heart. This can result in headache, swelling (possibly affecting the head, neck, and arms), difficulty breathing, or vision problems.

If bone marrow is involved, you may experience anemia that results in generalized weakness and **fatigue**. Bleeding may result from a low platelet count, or infections may occur as a result of a low white blood cell count. Occasionally, lymphoma can also involve the brain or spinal cord, resulting in headaches, double vision, or weakness in an arm or leg. With involvement of the spinal cord, back pain, leg weakness, numbness, or problems related to the control of bowel or bladder function may occur. Most commonly, the spinal cord itself is not involved, but the lymphoma may press on the spinal cord, resulting in these problems. If any symptoms of spinal cord involvement occur, you should see your doctor immediately or, at night, go to the emergency room, as any delay could result in paralysis.

Fatigue
tiredness, particularly the debilitating, continuous tiredness that signals illness or disease.

Other symptoms that can occur, regardless of the site of the lymphoma, may include fever, night sweats, and weight loss (these are the **B symptoms** that are mentioned in Question 19); when these symptoms are present to a significant degree, they indicate a more aggressive behaving lymphoma.

B symptoms
fevers, night sweats, and weight loss that may occur in lymphoma patients. They can occur individually or together.

Many people with lymphoma won't have any symptoms. In these cases, the enlarged lymph nodes may be felt in the shower or while lying in bed. Occasionally, your physician may detect them during a routine physical examination; this is more common with the **indolent** lymphomas.

Indolent
usually slow growing.

Another important point to remember is that no symptoms are unique to lymphoma. Most of the time, symptoms from something other than lymphoma will be seen. In most people with enlarged, painful lymph nodes, various infections are a much more common cause, but if the lymph node remains large or continues to grow, especially if it is not painful, you should see your physician, who should consider a biopsy.

11. How is lymphoma diagnosed?

The diagnosis of lymphoma is usually made from a lymph node biopsy. This involves obtaining an abnormal lymph node or a piece of an abnormal lymph node and examining it under a microscope. Before the biopsy, usually performed by a surgeon, your primary care doctor will have carried out a careful medical history, a physical examination, some blood tests, and perhaps some X-rays or scans.

Before the biopsy, usually performed by a surgeon, your primary care doctor will have carried out a careful medical history, a physical examination, some blood tests, and perhaps some X-rays or scans.

The biopsy can be an excisional biopsy in which the entire affected lymph node is removed, or an incisional biopsy in which only a small piece of a lymph node is removed. The surgeon will decide which type is best, depending on the location of the node. At certain locations, the smaller incisional biopsy may result in less risk of damage to normal structures such as blood vessels or nerves, while still providing adequate material for a diagnosis. The biopsy is usually performed in the doctor's office or in the hospital and, depending on which part of the body is involved, can be done with either a local or general anesthetic. Sometimes a needle alone is used to obtain a small sample of cells in a procedure called a **fine needle aspiration (FNA)**. This is easier to do and less

Fine needle aspiration (FNA)
a procedure to obtain a sample of tissue using a small needle.

invasive than either an excisional or incisional biopsy. However, for the purposes of diagnosing the lymphoma, it is generally not as good as taking out the entire lymph node, and, often, patients will need to undergo another procedure to obtain an adequate amount of tissue for a diagnosis. This is because when examining the cells under a microscope, it is important to see an overview of the pattern of how the cells appear (the bird's eye view) rather than just looking at the individual cells. This feature of the biopsy, termed the **lymph node architecture**, is often crucial when evaluating a lymph node for the possibility of lymphoma. Nevertheless, there are times when it is very hard to remove an entire lymph node, due to its particular location, or too many risks are involved in using a general anesthetic; thus, a fine needle aspiration may be adequate to make the diagnosis.

Lymph node architecture
the structure of lymph nodes when they are seen under a microscope.

After removal, the lymph node is sent to the laboratory, where the lymph node tissue is treated with special chemicals to "fix" it, which results in preservation of the tissue. Then it is cut into very thin sections, placed on glass slides, and stained, making it ready for the pathologist to examine. The staining allows the different cells and structures within the lymph node to be distinguished from one another.

The pathologist examines the lymph node to see whether the cells are normal or abnormal. It is common for lymph nodes to become enlarged in reaction to infection or inflammation, in which case the findings are **benign**. If it is **malignant**, it can be either lymphoma or a different type of cancer that has spread to the lymph node.

Benign
not cancerous.

Malignant
cancerous.

Flow cytometry
a procedure for examining the proteins present on the surface of cells.

Another helpful test, called **flow cytometry**, provides an additional way of examining and identifying different types of cells by looking at the pattern of particular proteins that exist on their surface. Different lymphomas have particular patterns of protein expression that help to determine the exact type of lymphoma. Flow cytometry will be performed in almost all cases in which lymphoma is suspected.

As you will see, given that there are so many different types of lymphoma and the differences between many of them can be very subtle, it can sometimes be very difficult to be sure of the type of lymphoma that one has. In these rare cases, it is a good idea to get a second opinion from another pathologist. This is especially true if knowing the exact type will change the way the lymphoma will be treated. In many cases, the difference is so subtle that it will not affect the treatment, and from a practical point of view, the distinction is less important.

12. Could my lymphoma have been diagnosed earlier, and does it make a difference?

When a lump is first discovered, depending on the circumstances and its characteristics, the internist or family doctor may want to keep an eye on the lump, as most lumps are due to benign causes and go away without treatment. In the vast majority of cases, the swelling may be due to infection or inflammation, and the doctor will prescribe antibiotics. Often, a biopsy will be considered only if the lump persists or has features suggesting the possibility of cancer.

However, if you find out that you have a lymphoma instead of an infection, it is natural to wonder why the diagnosis was not made sooner and whether the delay in diagnosis will have an effect on your outcome. Most doctors will not hesitate to discuss your concerns about the timing of the diagnosis; if this is not done, your questions may linger and distract you from coping with everything else that is happening. If all patients with a lump subsequently found not to be lymphoma were subjected to a biopsy, many unnecessary biopsies would be performed.

The question of whether diagnosing the lymphoma earlier makes a difference can be complicated. Lymphoma is very different from other cancers (such as breast, bowel, or lung cancer) in this respect. In these and other cancers, the ability to cure the disease largely depends on whether the cancer has spread from the site where it initially started. This is not generally true for lymphoma because the lymphatic system where the cancer begins is distributed throughout the body. Spreading from one place to another does not necessarily have the same ominous implications as it does in these other cancers. The ability to cure lymphoma depends more on what particular type of lymphoma you have—whether it is indolent or aggressive rather than whether it is in only one spot. That is not to say that having a lymphoma confined to one or two areas is not a better situation than having a lymphoma that is more widespread; nevertheless, lymphoma that has spread can also be cured.

13. What causes lymphoma?

The cause of lymphoma in most people remains unknown; it is easier, in fact, to list what doesn't cause lymphoma. No association has been made with smoking or alcohol use. Particular diets or lifestyles in general do not appear to increase the chance of developing lymphoma. Lymphoma does not occur as a result of previous injury, and it is not related to obesity. Lymphoma can't spread from one person to another. Based on the increased incidence in association with immunodeficiency or inflammation including autoimmune disorders, it is felt that chronic stimulation of lymphocytes plays a role in the development of lymphoma.

Acquired immunodeficiency syndrome (AIDS)

the syndrome resulting from infection with the human immunodeficiency virus (HIV).

It is very clear that an abnormal immune system increases the chances of developing lymphoma.

Human immunodeficiency virus (HIV)

a virus that attacks the human immune system, leaving the carrier prone to infections.

Many scientists have tried to identify certain things that could cause lymphoma. In most cases, the evidence for an association is weak, although exposure to certain chemicals such as insecticides or pesticides over prolonged periods of time may result in a higher incidence of lymphoma. These chemicals have been implicated in a higher incidence of non-Hodgkin's lymphoma among farm workers in some rural areas of the United States.

It is very clear that an abnormal immune system increases the chances of developing lymphoma. The most dramatic example of this is **acquired immunodeficiency syndrome (AIDS)**, caused by the **human immunodeficiency virus (HIV)**. This virus infects lymphocytes, resulting in depletion of CD4 helper cells. This results in a markedly abnormal immune system, which has been associated with a much higher incidence of lymphoma. Immune system abnormalities are also seen after heart, lung, kidney, or liver transplants, for which recipients are kept on drugs to prevent rejection, usually for the rest of their lives. These drugs inhibit the normal function of the lymphocytes and are associated with an increased incidence of lymphoma.

Autoimmune diseases can increase the risk of developing lymphoma. The most common associations occur with Sjogren's disease, autoimmune thyroiditis, and systemic lupus erythematosus. There does not appear to be a strong association with rheumatoid arthritis and the development of lymphoma. There is also not a strong association with inflammatory valve disease. The chronic stimulation that occurs in autoimmune disease or the immunosuppression that is given to treat the autoimmune disease can both be responsible for the increased risk of lymphoma.

Another virus that may cause lymphoma is the **Epstein-Barr virus**, which infects many people without causing illness and is also the cause of infectious mononucleosis (popularly known as "glandular fever" or "mono" and often called "the kissing disease," as it is common among adolescents and is spread through **saliva**). In the laboratory, this virus can make B lymphocytes grow abnormally. Some lymphoma patients have Epstein-Barr virus present in their lymphoma cells, suggesting that the virus may be involved in the development of their lymphoma; however, another explanation is that the immune abnormality that allowed the lymphoma to develop also allowed the Epstein-Barr virus infection to occur. This would make Epstein-Barr virus an innocent bystander infection rather than the cause of the lymphoma. Currently, the treatment of lymphoma is usually not different when Epstein-Barr virus is or is not present. Therefore, testing is not done on a routine basis. An exception to this is when lymphoma occurs after transplant, when testing for Epstein-Barr virus may be important.

Epstein-Barr virus

the virus that causes infectious mononucleosis and can cause lymphocytes to grow abnormally.

Saliva

the lubricating substance produced by the salivary glands that is essential for chewing and swallowing.

Hepatitis C virus
one of the viruses that can infect the liver and cause chronic liver inflammation.

Diffuse large B cell lymphoma
a type of intermediate-grade lymphoma.

The **hepatitis C virus** increases the chances of developing lymphoma. This is worrisome, as the number of people infected with this virus has increased dramatically over the past 20 years. Hepatitis C infection has been associated with the development of cryoglobulinemia, sometimes a precursor to lymphoma. It has also been associated with the development of aggressive lymphomas, including **diffuse large B cell lymphoma**. An association has not been found with follicular lymphoma.

Yet another virus that can cause lymphoma is the human herpes 8 virus. Another name for this virus is the Kaposi's sarcoma herpes virus. It has been associated with a particular type of lymphoma called primary effusion lymphoma. This is a lymphoma originally diagnosed in AIDS patients. It is occasionally seen in non-HIV-infected patients. It usually presents with fluid around the lung, heart, or in the abdominal cavity.

14. How is lymphoma classified?

Working Formulation
one of the lymphoma classifications.

Revised European-American Classification
the basis of the newest lymphoma classification.

World Health Organization Classification
associated with lymphoma classification

There are many different types of lymphoma. In order to make sense of the different types, a classification system is necessary. The fundamental classification is between Hodgkin's disease and non-Hodgkin's lymphoma. For non-Hodgkin's lymphomas, there have been a number of different classifications used over the years. These include the Rappaport, Kiel, Lukes-Collins, **Working Formulation**, **Revised European-American Classification**, and most recently, the **World Health Organization Classification**. The Working Formulation introduced in the early 1980s classified lymphomas into low grade, intermediate grade, and high grade based on the appearance of the lymphoma cells under the microscope. As a greater understanding of lymphoma has developed, and newer technology (flow cytometry) to evaluate proteins on the surface of lymphoma cells and genetic changes occurring within the cells has become available, a much greater ability to distinguish between similar types of lymphoma has emerged. This has resulted in the need for more sophisticated and helpful classification systems and ultimately led to the development of the World Health Organization classification. Appropriate classification is necessary for conducting **clinical trials**, where it is important to identify groups of patients with a similar type of lymphoma. This allows for the development and evaluation of treatments specifically geared toward the type of lymphoma studied.

Clinical trials
research studies evaluating promising new treatments in patients.

In the current World Health Organization classification, individual types of non-Hodgkin's lymphoma are listed according to a number of features, including the cell of origin (B cell, T cell, or NK cell). The appearance of the lymphoma under the microscope, the types of protein present on the surface of the cells, genetic features, and clinical behavior were all considered. It is useful in clinical practice to consider groups of these entities according to whether they behave in an indolent fashion or an aggressive fashion. All this information is then used to determine the appropriate type of treatment, or if one is considering a clinical trial option, ensuring that appropriate patients are enrolled into that clinical trial.

For Hodgkin's lymphoma, there are two broad categories. These include classical Hodgkin's lymphoma and nodular lymphocyte predominant Hodgkin's lymphoma.

15. How is lymphoma staged?

Stage
a reference to the number of places in the body affected by lymphoma or other cancer.

There are four possible **stages** (see Table 3) based on the extent of the lymphoma throughout the body and whether there is involvement of organs outside the lymph node system. Each stage can be further divided into A or B, depending on whether significant B symptoms, which include fever, night sweats, and weight loss, have been present (see Question 10 for more on symptoms). In general, the presence of B symptoms suggests that the lymphoma is more aggressive.

Ann Arbor Staging System
used to describe the areas in the body affected by the lymphoma. It was created at a conference held in Ann Arbor, Michigan.

A group of lymphoma experts (meeting in Ann Arbor, Michigan, in 1971) devised the staging system that is known as the **Ann Arbor Staging System**. Since then, it has been applied very successfully to non-Hodgkin's lymphoma and remains the best staging system available for non-Hodgkin's lymphoma.

Staging is very important information for every patient with lymphoma, as it provides a common language for doctors and patients to describe the areas affected

Table 3 Staging of lymphoma*

Stage I	One lymph node area involved
Stage II	Two or more lymph node areas on the *same side* of the diaphragm
Stage III	Lymph nodes involved on *both sides* of the diaphragm
Stage IV	Any of the above with involvement of sites other than lymph nodes (most commonly the bone marrow, liver, or lungs)
B symptoms	Fever, night sweats, or significant weight loss

*After designation of the stage based on the sites of involvement, patients are categorized as either A (if no B symptoms are present) or B (if B symptoms are present).

within the body and its overall extent. The same staging system is used for all lymphomas, regardless of whether it is an indolent or aggressive type. It is vital information for deciding on the correct treatment and can also be helpful in estimating **prognosis**.

Prognosis
a prediction of the course that a disease will take.

As noted, there are four stages described in the Ann Arbor system (the staging system uses Roman numerals). In this way, lymphoma can be designated as "limited" for stages I and II and "more extensive" for stages III and IV.

Stage I refers to involvement of a single lymph node region. Stage II refers to two or more lymph node regions, with the affected regions occurring on the same side of the **diaphragm** (the large muscle that separates the chest from the abdomen and is important for breathing). Stage III is where lymph node regions are involved on both sides of the diaphragm. (For the purposes of staging, the spleen is included as a lymph node region.) Stage IV includes involvement of disease not only in lymph node regions, but also in non–lymph node sites such as the bone marrow, liver, lungs, gut, or skin.

Diaphragm
the large muscle that separates the lungs from the abdomen. Its movement is important for breathing.

The presence of lymphoma involving a site other than the lymph nodes or spleen generally implies stage IV unless the involvement is from direct spread from a lymph node. For example, if there is involvement of the lung directly next to involved lymph nodes in the chest, the subscript E is written beside the stage. Thus, III_E would indicate that lymph nodes on both sides of the diaphragm are involved and that lymphoma has extended out from a lymph node into a surrounding organ. Stage IV refers to lymphoma involving a nonlymphoid organ such as the bone marrow, liver, or lung where it is not directly spreading from a lymph node.

Until about 15 years ago, many people with lymphoma underwent a surgical procedure called a **laparotomy** for staging. This procedure involved opening the abdomen, taking samples or biopsies of many lymph nodes, performing a liver biopsy, and removing the spleen. The spleen, lymph node, and liver biopsies would then be examined under a microscope to determine whether there was involvement by lymphoma.

Laparotomy

surgery involving an incision to look directly into the abdomen.

The laparotomy was necessary because **computed tomography (CT) scans** done to look for lymphoma in the liver or spleen can be normal unless these organs are enlarged. A normal-sized liver or spleen may still be involved with lymphoma and may appear entirely normal on a scan. In such cases, the only way to tell was to do a surgical biopsy; however, because this was major surgery, it was only performed if absolutely necessary for treatment planning to know whether the lymphoma was limited (stage I or stage II) or more extensive (stage III or stage IV). Nowadays, with improved imaging methods and treatment and other ways to predict involvement in the liver and spleen, this surgery is rarely performed.

Computed tomography (CT) scan

a specialized type of X-ray that creates a detailed cross-sectional view of the body.

Staging now relies on a physical examination, X-rays, CT scans, and bone marrow examination. **Positron emission tomography (PET)** scanning is also useful (Table 4).

Positron emission tomography (PET)

X-ray studies that use the abnormal sugar metabolism of cancer cells to identify metastatic deposits.

The physical examination for staging focuses on determining whether there is enlargement of the lymph nodes, liver, and spleen. On examination, enlarged lymph nodes in the head and neck region, the armpit (axilla), and also the groin can be detected. Lymph nodes are occasionally felt in the elbow or knee region. In order for the spleen to be felt, it needs to be two

Table 4 Tests for staging of lymphoma

Tests necessary for staging	Tests sometimes required
Physical examination	CT scan of neck and chest
Chest X-ray	PET scan
CT scan of abdomen and pelvis	Bone marrow biopsy on both sides
Bone marrow biopsy	Gallium scan
	Spinal tap

to three times larger than normal. Radiologic studies (X-ray, CT, or **magnetic resonance imaging** [MRI]) are needed to detect lymph node enlargement internally that cannot be felt on examination. These include the lymph nodes between the lungs (hilar and **mediastinal nodes**) and the lymph nodes in the abdomen (**retroperitoneal** and **mesenteric lymph nodes**). In people without lymphoma, lymph nodes are normally present at these sites but are not enlarged, usually measuring up to only 1 cm.

Magnetic resonance imaging
a technique based on the use of magnetic fields to produce images of body parts.

Mediastinal nodes
lymph nodes present in the area between the lungs.

Retroperitoneal lymph nodes
the most common lymph nodes present in the abdomen.

Mesenteric lymph nodes
the lymph nodes present in the abdomen tissue that anchors the bowel.

The most commonly used radiologic test for staging is the CT scan (also known as a CAT scan). The X-ray camera takes many individual pictures at different angles, and these are then combined into multiple, computer-generated, cross-sectional images at each level that needs to be examined. Often, scans are obtained of the chest, abdomen, and pelvis. Many physicians will obtain a CT scan of the abdomen and pelvis only and will use a plain X-ray of the chest to evaluate the lymph nodes above the diaphragm. The plain X-ray of the chest often gives as much information for staging as the CT scan. A CT scan of the neck can be obtained if there is doubt about involvement of

The most commonly used radiologic test for staging is the CT scan (also known as a CAT scan).

the neck lymph nodes. MRI scans can also be used for staging and may be useful instead of a CT scan under special circumstances. In order to get the best CT scan pictures, **contrast dye** is given orally and intravenously. The dye allows better visualization between the lymph nodes and other tissues, including blood vessels and gut; however, the dye can occasionally affect kidney function. If your doctor feels that you are at risk for this side effect, an MRI can be used instead of a CT scan. The contrast dye can also cause allergic reactions that require premedication with a small dose of steroids before the CT scan. CT and MRI scans are very good for examining the size of lymph nodes but do not tell you definitively whether big lymph nodes contain lymphoma. At the time of diagnosis, if a lymph node biopsy confirms lymphoma, it is reasonable to assume that other big lymph nodes are also involved with lymphoma; however, after treatment, lymph nodes can remain enlarged due to large amounts of inflammation or scar tissue. These nodes will still look big on a CT or MRI scan. It is important in this situation to be able to tell the difference between big lymph nodes caused by active lymphoma versus big nodes resulting from scar tissue. Another biopsy is the only way to be absolutely sure; however, a PET scan may also be very helpful. The PET scan involves injection of a radioactive tracer into the bloodstream. Active lymphoma cells pick up the tracer, and, therefore, even if the lymph nodes are not enlarged, areas of lymphoma can still be detected with a positron camera. A PET scan can also be useful for staging lymphoma when it is first diagnosed.

Contrast dye

a chemical that is injected for certain X-rays, including CT scans and MRI scans, that results in better contrast pictures.

Although a **lymphangiogram** is an older test that is rarely done nowadays, as it is technically a difficult test for the radiologist to perform, it has been used for staging. Because it is rarely done, few radiologists have much experience in either performing or interpreting the test. The procedure involves injecting dye into the lymph vessels of both feet. These vessels are very tiny and difficult to find. Once injected, the dye travels to the lymph nodes in the groin and abdomen and can show abnormal lymph nodes even if they are not larger than normal.

Lymphangiogram
an X-ray study of lymph glands after they are injected with a dye.

A **gallium scan**, another test that can be used for staging, involves giving a small amount of radioactive gallium as an intravenous injection. After the injection, scanning is performed 2 and 3 days later. Some lymphomas take up the gallium, whereas others do not. In order to know whether a gallium scan will be useful, a baseline scan needs to be obtained before treatment. This scan tells you whether your lymphoma takes up gallium; if so, additional gallium scans will be useful to follow the response to treatment. Similar to the PET scan, the gallium scan can be useful to evaluate enlarged lymph nodes that persist after treatment, helping to differentiate between scar tissue and active lymphoma.

Gallium scan
a nuclear medicine test that uses gallium to show areas of lymphoma within the body.

A bone marrow examination is also part of the staging evaluation. Occasionally, it is important to do this test on both sides of the hipbone (a bilateral biopsy).

Lymphoma staging is important primarily to identify patients who have limited stage disease, and therefore may benefit from a different treatment approach than patients with more extensive disease.

16. How is a bone marrow examination performed?

Evaluation of the bone marrow is a routine part of lymphoma staging. When bone marrow involvement occurs, production of all the normal blood cells may be decreased, resulting in a low red cell count (anemia), a low platelet count (**thrombocytopenia**), or a low white cell count (**leukopenia**). If there is lymphoma involvement in the bone marrow, the lymphoma is stage IV.

Thrombocytopenia
a low platelet count.

Leukopenia
a low white blood cell count.

When staging lymphoma for the first time, a bone marrow sample may be obtained from both sides of the hip because only one side may contain the lymphoma. Bone marrow sampling is important, as it affects the choice of treatment and is also frequently necessary for evaluating the response to treatment.

Bone marrow sampling is important, as it affects the choice of treatment and is also frequently necessary for evaluating the response to treatment.

The bone marrow is obtained from the hipbone at the back, generally at the site of the **dimples of Venus**, next to the tailbone. This procedure, usually done in 20 to 30 minutes in the outpatient clinic, can be done with the patient lying on either his or her side or front. The bone marrow test has two parts: bone marrow aspiration, which refers to the sampling of the liquid part of the bone marrow within the marrow cavity, and bone marrow biopsy, which involves taking a tiny core of the bone that, when looked at under the microscope, shows the bird's eye view of the marrow within the bone.

Dimples of Venus
the dimples seen on the skin over the sacrum on the lower back.

First, the skin over the site on the hipbone is cleansed with a disinfectant and then numbed with local anesthetic, usually lidocaine. Next, the area down to the surface of the bone is numbed. The surface of the bone can be particularly sensitive when the lidocaine is first injected, as the lidocaine causes a stinging sensation. Next, a very small incision is made. The bone marrow needle is then drilled into the marrow cavity with a gentle corkscrew type of motion, which usually causes a pressure. The inside of the bone marrow is liquid, and a small amount (2 to 5 cc) is then sucked out with the needle. This only takes a couple of seconds, but for many people it is the worst part of the procedure. The bone marrow itself cannot be anesthetized, and when it is sucked out it can feel like a very strange pulling sensation in the hip and also down the leg. The person doing the procedure can help by talking to you, describing each step, and giving you a warning before the marrow is withdrawn. This discomfort should only last a couple of seconds.

The second part of the test involves doing the biopsy. The biopsy needle is placed in the same area on the hipbone, and a hollow needle is drilled into the bone. Again, this should feel only like a pressure sensation. The needle is then removed with the piece of bone inside. Pressure is held over the site to prevent bleeding, and a bandage is applied to the area. This is the end of the procedure.

17. How do I prepare for a bone marrow test?

For many people, the worst part of the test is waiting for the appointment. The build-up of anxiety may actually increase the pain and discomfort associated with the test. Thus, a shorter appointment time may be helpful. If you are taking aspirin or a similar type of drug that prevents platelets from working properly, ask your doctor whether it should be stopped. Many patients find it helpful to have a friend or relative accompany them to the appointment. Usually a sedative is not necessary for the procedure, so patients can drive themselves to and from the appointment if necessary. In fact, many patients return to work after the test.

After the test, you can be up and about as normal. You may feel some aching discomfort in the area of the biopsy after the local anesthetic wears off, but this should only last for 1 or 2 days. A mild over-the-counter painkiller is usually effective in controlling the discomfort. Aspirin or similar medications are to be avoided, as they can increase the chance of bleeding. Bleeding from the site of the biopsy can occur, and simply applying pressure will generally stop most bleeding. It is very rare for an infection or serious bleeding to result from a bone marrow test.

18. What are the different types of non-Hodgkin's lymphoma?

The individual types of lymphoma are classified as either indolent or aggressive.

Indolent non-Hodgkin's lymphoma

Indolent lymphomas generally are slow growing, and their appearance under the microscope provides the diagnosis. These lymphomas tend to grow slowly and respond well to therapy, often initially obtaining long periods of remission, but eventually the lymphoma tends to recur. The indolent non-Hodgkin's lymphomas are generally considered incurable. At the time of diagnosis, the lymphoma is often stage 4, when bone marrow and lymph node areas are usually involved.

Circulating lymphoma cells may be seen in the bloodstream, and patients often have no symptoms.

Aggressive non-Hodgkin's lymphoma

Aggressive non-Hodgkin's lymphoma includes the group of lymphomas previously termed intermediate-grade lymphomas and also high-grade lymphomas. These lymphomas grow faster than the indolent lymphomas. They generally cause symptoms more rapidly and require the prompt institution of therapy. Most cases will present as stage I or II. This is in contrast to the indolent lymphomas, which frequently present as stage IV. Involvement of tissues or organs other than lymph nodes is also more common in this category of lymphoma.

19. What is small lymphocytic lymphoma/chronic lymphocytic leukemia?

Small lymphocytic lymphoma (SLL) is very closely related to a type of chronic leukemia called **chronic lymphocytic leukemia**, or CLL. These disorders are so closely associated that they are grouped together in the current World Health Organization **lymphoma classification**. The "small" in the name refers to the size of the lymphoma cells when seen under the microscope. This is generally a slow-growing lymphoma that occurs mostly in older people. At diagnosis, lymphoma involving the bone marrow is common, and most people are therefore in stage IV. The difference between the two diseases really depends on how many of the abnormal cells are present in the blood as compared with the lymph nodes. When the cells are most

Small lymphocytic lymphoma

a type of indolent lymphoma that is similar to chronic lymphocytic leukemia.

Chronic lymphocytic leukemia

the most common slow-growing type of leukemia.

Lymphoma classification

a system to organize the many different types of lymphoma.

abundant in the blood, it is called CLL. Although CLL is relatively common, this type of lymphoma is relatively rare, accounting for less than 5% of all non-Hodgkin's lymphomas. The abnormal lymph nodes and blood both contain mature B lymphocytes. It is unusual to have disease confined to the lymph nodes. Most patients will also have abnormal lymphocytes in the circulation. SLL is usually diagnosed after small, slowly growing lymph nodes are found. An abnormal blood test with a high white count consisting mostly of lymphocytes may also lead to the diagnosis. B symptoms are unusual. General management of **follicular lymphomas** is discussed in Question 20. Similar principles apply to SLL.

Follicular lymphomas

lymphomas composed of lymphocytes organized into round structures.

20. What is follicular lymphoma—grade 1 and 2?

Grade 1 and 2 follicular lymphomas are the most common of the non-Hodgkin's lymphomas. The specific type of lymphoma is determined by the number of large cells present among the small lymphocytes (small cleaved cells) that make up the bulk of the lymphoma cells. More is understood about the abnormalities that occur in the lymphocytes leading to this type of lymphoma than in many other lymphomas. A hallmark of this type of lymphoma is the presence of too much of a protein called Bcl-2. A gene called bcl-2 produces this protein, and the excess Bcl-2 allows the lymphocyte to live longer than is normal. Because the abnormal lymphocytes fail to die, which happens during normal cell turnover, too many lymphocytes accumulate, eventually forming lymph node tumors. The reason for the overproduction of Bcl-2 is also understood. All humans have 23 pairs of chromosomes—46 chromosomes in all—that contain many, many genes. The genes are made up of **deoxyribonucleic acid (DNA)**, and each contains the fundamental information necessary for the manufacture of a protein. The process responsible for making a protein from the message contained in a gene is normally regulated very closely in order to prevent too much of a protein being produced. Sometimes genes can get moved from one chromosome to another; such an event is called **translocation**. In the follicular lymphomas, the gene for the production of the Bcl-2 protein gets moved from chromosome 18 to chromosome 14. On chromosome 14, bcl-2 is placed next to another gene that gives it instructions to keep producing the Bcl-2 protein. As mentioned previously, the Bcl-2 protein prevents the lymphocyte from dying at the right time. Normal lymphocytes are programmed to die at the end of their normal life span. This built-in death program is called **apoptosis** (programmed cell death) and is essentially a cell suicide program. If this process is blocked (e.g., by having too much Bcl-2), lymphocytes accumulate, and lymphoma may result. Many chemotherapy drugs that are useful in lymphoma act by causing lymphocytes to undergo programmed cell death, but when too much Bcl-2 is present, the lymphoma can be more resistant to chemotherapy. Clinical trials evaluating compounds that could be given to patients to specifically block the Bcl-2 protein from performing its normal function are ongoing. The hope is that this will then allow cells to die normally and also to respond better to chemotherapy. It appears that monoclonal antibodies act partly through activation of cell death pathways. In October 2002, the Nobel

Deoxyribonucleic acid (DNA)
the material that carries the genetic code for each organism or person.

Translocation
an abnormality of certain chromosomes seen in some cancer cells.

Apoptosis
a process by which normal cells die. Some cancer cells do not die, and a failure of cells to undergo apoptosis can contribute to the growth of cancer. It is often referred to as "programmed cell death."

Prize for medicine was awarded to researchers who discovered the basics of this important cell suicide program.

The average age at which this type of lymphoma occurs is 55 to 60 years. Males and females are equally affected. Approximately half the patients with stage IV lymphoma will have B symptoms (fevers, night sweats, and weight loss), but the symptoms occur much less frequently in patients with stage I to stage III disease.

Often, the first noticeable symptom is a lump in the neck or groin that may have been present for a while and that is usually painless. It is common for the lymph node swelling to vary in size over time, maybe even getting smaller (waxing and waning). A biopsy is needed for diagnosis, and it is best if the pathologist removes the entire lymph node (an excisional biopsy) for examination. The pathologist will be more likely to be sure of the diagnosis if more of the node is available. Removing the entire lymph node does not help in treatment, except possibly in the very unlikely event that it is the only site involved (stage I disease). Some doctors may first suggest doing a needle aspiration (putting a needle into the enlarged lymph node and sucking out some cells into a syringe), as this may be sufficient in some cases. The cells are then sent to the pathologist, who examines them under the microscope. Unfortunately, because the pathologist is unable to see the bird's eye view but only the individual cells, it is generally not possible to tell whether there are **follicles** or nodules (referred to as the architecture of the lymph node), and an excisional biopsy will often be needed in addition.

Follicles

round structures containing lymphocytes.

In some cases, the only enlarged lymph nodes may not be easy to biopsy. Examples include lymph nodes deep inside the chest, between the lungs, or inside the abdomen. In these cases, needle aspirations may be all that are possible. A laparoscopic biopsy (keyhole surgery) can sometimes be performed to obtain a larger piece of the lymph node.

You will be referred to a **hematologist/oncologist** after a diagnosis is made. At that point, staging tests are performed, and decisions about treatment are discussed.

Hematologist/oncologist
a physician specializing in the treatment of blood disorders and cancer.

21. What is follicular grade 3 non-Hodgkin's lymphoma?

Follicular lymphomas are currently divided into three groups. These are grade 1, grade 2, and grade 3. Grade 3 has more recently been divided into grade 3A and grade 3B. Both grades 1 and 2 lymphomas are generally considered to be indolent lymphomas, whereas grade 3 is considered to be an aggressive lymphoma. In reality, grade 3A may behave more like the indolent lymphomas and grade 3B more like an aggressive lymphoma. Unfortunately, this situation is more complicated, as the ability of most pathologists to distinguish between grade 3A and 3B and even between grade 2 and grade 3 is often not very good. This is based on studies showing that when the same biopsy is looked at by different pathologists, they frequently disagree on the grade.

Grade 3 lymphomas are the least common of the follicular lymphomas. Staging of these lymphomas is the same as for other types of non-Hodgkin's lymphoma, and the treatment is similar to that of either other indolent follicular non-Hodgkin's lymphomas or diffuse large B cell lymphoma (see Question 22), depending on the specific grade and patient-related features.

In practice, because the difference between grade 3A and 3B is difficult to determine, most patients are just classified as grade 3. The treatment is most commonly chemotherapy plus an anti-CD20 monoclonal antibody. This is similar to the treatment usually given to patients with diffuse large B cell lymphoma. Long-term remissions are the goal of treatment and the belief of a lower incidence of relapse with grade 3B versus grade 3A is now being questioned.

22. What is diffuse large B cell lymphoma?

Diffuse large B cell lymphoma (DLBCL) is one of the most common types of lymphoma. It accounts for approximately 30–40% of all cases of lymphoma. DLBCL occurs mostly in adults of middle age and older but is also not uncommon in younger individuals. The average age at which patients develop this type of lymphoma is 60 years. Many cases are curable with chemotherapy, but if they are not treated, the lymphoma usually grows rapidly and can result in death within a year. Most of these lymphomas arise from B lymphocytes, but 25% arise from T cells.

One-third of these lymphomas are localized when first diagnosed. The occurrence of the lymphoma at sites other than the lymph nodes, including the bone marrow, gut, lungs, kidneys, and liver, is not uncommon.

Often, the first symptom noted may be a rapidly growing lump that is generally painless, but tenderness may be noted because the capsule of the lymph node gets stretched rapidly. Initially, patients may be given antibiotics to treat a suspected infection, as this is a more likely cause of lymph node swelling. If the lymph node does not return to normal over a few weeks with or without antibiotics, a lymph node biopsy should be obtained. Abdominal pain or discomfort, cough, shortness of breath, or a sensation of fullness in the chest or neck may also be the first abnormality noted. Fevers and night sweats may occur, and weight loss may also be noted (these are the B symptoms).

PART THREE

Staging and Treatment of Lymphoma

What happens after I'm told that I have lymphoma?

Should I get a second opinion?

Apart from the biopsy, what other information is needed?

More . . .

23. What happens after I'm told that I have lymphoma?

Hearing that you have lymphoma, as with any form of serious illness or cancer, can be a frightening and overwhelming experience. For most people, it is the first serious illness that they have faced, and many different emotions may arise. Patients often experience the various stages that are commonly associated with the grieving process, namely denial, anger, bargaining, **depression**, and finally acceptance. The duration and intensity of the different stages vary among individuals.

Depression
a disorder characterized by excessive sadness and feelings of hopelessness.

The surgeon who performed the biopsy is the first person to receive the results, which will be discussed with you at your first follow-up visit; however, many surgeons may not feel comfortable addressing the multitude of questions that are foremost in your mind. An appointment will be arranged with a lymphoma specialist, who can provide you with some answers. Whenever possible, this appointment should take place sooner rather than later so that your questions can be answered to help minimize your anxiety and fears.

Hematology
the study of diseases of the blood, including blood cancers.

Oncology
the field of medicine that studies cancer.

A lymphoma specialist is a physician who is trained in **hematology** or **oncology**—and frequently both of these specialties. A hematologist has received specialty training in the management of blood disorders, including cancers related to the blood and lymphatic systems, such as lymphoma, leukemia, and multiple myeloma. An oncologist is a specialist who is trained in the management of all cancers in general. Most hematology and oncology training programs in the

United States are combined, and as a result, most lymphoma patients receive treatment from a physician trained in both of these specialties. In communities with a university teaching hospital, there are often groups of physicians who specialize in mainly lymphoma or mainly leukemia.

The first step in coming to terms with the diagnosis is arming yourself with information and deciding on a plan of management. Therefore, hopefully, your appointment with the lymphoma specialist can be expedited. For the first appointment, it is a good idea to bring your spouse, a close relative, or a friend to provide much-needed emotional support, to remember to ask helpful questions, and to help in remembering the details. You may also find it helpful to tape record the meeting, as a lot of information can be discussed at that first appointment. Before your appointment, your primary care doctor or surgeon will generally send or fax your medical records, including the biopsy results, to the lymphoma specialist's office. This allows your lymphoma doctor to review your information before the meeting. The benefit is that more time from the appointment can be dedicated to discussion about the nature of lymphoma, what other tests are needed, and how best to treat the disease. Your specialist will wish to review the symptoms that you have been experiencing and also obtain additional information about your past medical history. Because you have likely told the same story to a number of doctors and nurses previously, this can seem very repetitive; however, to ensure that nothing gets missed, this process is very important and is usually time well spent for both you and your new physician. This allows you and your doctor to get to know each other better.

At the initial visit, you may first meet with a nurse or medical assistant who will obtain some baseline information. After filling out a form that provides details of your past medical and surgical history, family history, medications, and any drug allergies, you then will meet with the lymphoma doctor, who will ask questions about your symptoms and how you are currently feeling. You will then change into a gown to be examined. Gynecologic and rectal examinations are usually not required. The most important parts of the examination are the lymph nodes, liver, and spleen, but a general examination is also important in evaluating any other areas that the lymphoma may be affecting and what these effects might be, and also to get a sense of your overall health. This information is vital for deciding on the appropriate treatment. You may or may not prefer having your friend or relative remain in the room during the appointment or examination.

The most important parts of the examination are the lymph nodes, liver, and spleen, but a general examination is also important in evaluating any other areas that the lymphoma may be affecting and what these effects might be, and also to get a sense of your overall health.

After the examination, your doctor will discuss lymphoma in general and your lymphoma in particular. Other required tests, including blood tests, scans, and usually a bone marrow examination, will give a complete picture of the extent of the lymphoma. A full discussion of the stage of the lymphoma and a treatment plan may need to wait for the next visit after the tests are completed. At that time, enough information will be available to allow for a more detailed discussion of your particular lymphoma. If possible, it is better not to discuss too much information at that first visit, especially if you are hearing the diagnosis for the first time. At the time of the next visit, your thinking can be much clearer, and you'll be able to absorb a lot more information. Your doctor may also be able to provide you with some reading material relating to lymphoma or to useful websites on the Internet.

24. Should I get a second opinion?

A second opinion is a good idea if there is any doubt regarding the correct diagnosis, if you have any concerns about the proposed treatment, or if you do not feel good about your first lymphoma doctor. If there is doubt regarding the diagnosis, you may request that another pathologist review the slides. In most cases, however, as long as adequate material has been obtained for review by the pathologist, the diagnosis is not in doubt, and often more than one pathologist within the department has already examined the slides. It can be comforting, however, to receive confirmation of the diagnosis and treatment options from another lymphoma specialist. Sometimes seeking a second opinion may result in transferring your care to the new doctor, depending on your preference and the options that your insurance company will allow. In any event, your first lymphoma doctor should be comfortable in having you seek a second opinion if you wish. Usually, his or her office will give you a copy of all relevant material, including clinic notes and reports from the lymph node and bone marrow biopsies and any radiology studies, such as CT and PET scans. The doctor who provides the second opinion will require these reports and will probably also need to have the actual biopsy slides and X-rays evaluated at the hospital to ensure that the advice given is based on accurate information.

It is important to recognize that there are many acceptable options and often more than one correct option for dealing with a diagnosis of lymphoma. You may, therefore, receive different recommendations from different physicians, with none of them being wrong. Some patients may then seek a third opinion, getting yet another set of recommendations. If you feel comfortable with your first physician and all of your questions have been answered satisfactorily, second opinions may really be unnecessary and may lead to delays in proceeding with treatment as you attempt to sort all of the different options.

25. Apart from the biopsy, what other information is needed?

As mentioned previously, after the first time you see your lymphoma specialist, additional tests will need to be performed. These tests are needed to determine the answers to several questions. First, what is the stage of your lymphoma? This relates to which body parts are affected. CT scans to examine the lymph nodes in the chest, abdomen, and pelvis are required. A CT scan of the neck may also be obtained. A bone marrow biopsy is performed to evaluate the lymphoma at that site. Sometimes a bone marrow biopsy will be performed on both hips if the information makes a difference for treatment. A PET scan may also be obtained, as it may provide additional information in some cases of lymphoma. Other tests performed less frequently include an MRI or a gallium scan. These tests are discussed in Question 15 and can provide important information in some cases. Other tests are performed to provide information on how your particular lymphoma is likely to behave over time—in other words, to determine the likely prognosis. Question 18 describes how, in general, indolent lymphomas can be quite slow growing and can be managed with intermittent treatment over fairly long periods of time; however, while this is true in the average patient with indolent lymphoma, there may be certain features specific to you that give a better idea of whether your lymphoma will be more or less aggressive. The features that are useful for determining the prognosis have been pooled together into prognostic indices. For indolent lymphoma, the **Follicular Lymphoma International Prognostic Index (FLIPI)** is used. For aggressive lymphomas, the **International Prognostic Index (IPI)** is used. (Question 26). All of this information can be obtained from the scans, blood tests, and bone marrow examination.

Follicular Lymphoma International Prognostic Index (FLIPI)
a modified form of the IPI for determining the prognosis of patients with follicular lymphomas.

International Prognostic Index (IPI)
a system to determine the prognosis of patients with lymphoma.

Other information needed will depend on your general health apart from the lymphoma. This information is important in determining your ability to tolerate the various treatment options. For example, your doctor may need to evaluate how well your heart is functioning, as some chemotherapy drugs used to treat lymphoma can affect heart function. If there is any concern about the ability of your heart to tolerate that treatment, an alternative chemotherapy drug may be chosen. Similarly, special breathing tests, called **pulmonary function tests**, may be required, as some drugs can cause lung damage. This damage may be worsened if your lung function is not optimal before beginning chemotherapy.

Pulmonary function tests
a set of tests performed to evaluate the ability of the lungs to function properly.

All of this information is generally obtained before starting treatment for the lymphoma. After the test results are available, your doctor will schedule another appointment to discuss the results and treatment plan with you.

26. What is the IPI?

The International Prognostic Index (IPI) is a method that is used to estimate a statistical chance of how well you will do with treatment. It was first introduced for intermediate-grade lymphoma but appears to be useful for many other types of non-Hodgkin's lymphomas also. First introduced in 1993, it has gained wide acceptance but is limited in terms of its ability to be useful in planning treatment of lymphoma. In large studies from the United States, Canada, and Europe, a number of features of the patients' lymphoma were documented and then correlated with the results of treatment. Certain of these features, when combined, allowed separation of patients into better and poorer prognosis groups. Another group with an intermediate prognosis was also identified.

Lactate dehydrogenase

an enzyme measured using a simple blood test.

Performance status

the level of ability with which patients can perform their routine daily activities.

Central nervous system

the brain and spinal cord.

The following features helpful for determining prognosis were combined into this IPI: (1) age, (2) stage, (3) serum **lactate dehydrogenase** (LDH), (4) **performance status**, and (5) extranodal involvement. These features require further explanation. Older patients in general fare worse than younger ones; therefore, an age older than 60 receives one point in the index. Second, patients with stage I or stage II disease generally do better than patients with stage III or stage IV disease; therefore, stage III or stage IV disease receives another point. The third feature is the level of LDH in the bloodstream. LDH is present in red blood cells, liver, bone, and many other tissues. It is frequently increased in lymphoma patients and reflects the size of lymphoma and the rate at which it is growing. A level above normal is an additional risk factor and receives another point. Another point is given if the lymphoma involves sites other than the lymph nodes, including the bone marrow, the gut, liver, lung, and **central nervous system** (including the brain and spinal cord). The final feature in the IPI is the performance status, which is a measure of how well one is able to carry out one's everyday activities. The Eastern Cooperative Oncology Group scale is shown in Table 5.

Other scoring systems, such as the **Karnofsky Performance Status scale**, are also used to evaluate the level of functioning.

Karnofsky Performance Status scale
a system to evaluate how patients do when performing normal daily activities.

Thus, because there are five features in the IPI, any patient can have a score of 0 to 5, but most patients have a score of between 0 and 3. The score allows your doctor to estimate your likely response to treatment. The likelihood of success of the therapy is greatest with a lower score. Patients with higher scores may also do very well, as these likelihoods are statistical and may not apply to individual patients. If you are younger than age 60, the presence of lymphoma in sites other than the lymph nodes doesn't result in a worse prognosis. As a result, a modification to the IPI was made,

Table 5 Eastern Cooperative Oncology Group Performance Status Scale

0	No symptoms; fully active; able to carry out all normal activities.
1	Symptoms present but able to carry out normal activities; some difficulty with more strenuous activities.
2	Able to carry out normal self-care activities but limited in ability to work; up and about more than 50% of the time.
3	Capable of only limited self-care; confined to bed or chair more than 50% of waking hours.
4	Completely disabled; needing full-time assistance with normal self-care activities.

resulting in the age-adjusted IPI. This relies on only three factors to determine the prognosis: stage, lactate dehydrogenase, and the performance status.

An example of how this information is important relates to decisions regarding treatment. If you have a higher score on the IPI, you may wish to consider other treatments that may be available only through participation in a clinical trial. The IPI is also useful to ensure that patients being treated in a clinical trial where two treatments are being compared have similar characteristics. This ensures that any difference found between the two treatments is related to the treatment and not to differences in the patients who were treated in each group. It is important to realize that the IPI was developed for the intermediate-grade lymphomas.

Another problem with the IPI is that it was developed from evaluation of patients treated before anti-CD20 monoclonal antibodies were available for the treatment of lymphoma. As a result, the group from the University of British Columbia at Vancouver has reported on a revised international prognostic index that may become more generally accepted in the future for patients with aggressive lymphoma who received a particular monoclonal antibody combined with chemotherapy.

27. What is the FLIPI?

The prognostic index specific to follicular lymphomas, the Follicular Lymphoma International Prognostic Index (FLIPI) is similar to the IPI and is used to estimate prognosis for indolent lymphomas. Like the IPI, it has also gained widespread acceptance. The IPI was somewhat helpful when deciding on prognoses for indolent lymphoma patients but did not discriminate groups with differing outcomes as well as the FLIPI. It is not particularly helpful for deciding whether someone needs to commence therapy or deciding on a specific type of therapy, and, similar to the IPI, FLIPI is more useful for interpreting the results of large clinical studies. It can, however, be helpful to patients in considering their treatment options and outlook.

As with the IPI, the FLIPI includes five diagnostic criteria. However, the FLIPI adapts these criteria to reflect the specific features known to affect the prognosis in follicular lymphoma. These criteria include: (1) more than four nodal areas, (2) elevated serum lactate dehydrogenase levels, (3) age older than 60 years, (4) stage III or IV, and (5) anemia defined as a hemoglobin less than 12 g/dL. Scoring is performed in the same manner as with the IPI, with a score of 0–1 being considered low risk and a score of 3–5 being considered higher risk.

With improvements in chemotherapy regimens, differences between patients may not be so great, and, therefore, the IPI and FLIPI may become less useful. One final note about these scores and prognostic indicators: You must always remember that they are an estimate of how you might respond given your circumstances, and they should be considered in determining how to manage your particular lymphoma and your long-term prognosis but cannot be used to decide on any particular treatment plan. They do not in any way predict the future, nor are they a statistic that dooms you to certain death or certain recovery. Patients with a poor prognosis according to these indicators often do survive lymphoma. It is important that you do not give up

One final note about these scores and prognostic indicators: You must always remember that they are an estimate of how you might respond given your circumstances, and they should be considered in determining how to manage your particular lymphoma and your long-term prognosis but cannot be used to decide on any particular treatment plan.

simply because you're facing a more daunting life-threatening challenge. Some of the more aggressive lymphomas are also some of the most curable types of cancer. Survival depends a great deal on determination to take your treatment seriously and to work hard to maintain and improve your health status. On the other hand, patients with a good prognosis could misinterpret this estimate as a guarantee of survival; if they do not pay close attention to their treatment regimen and overall health, they could find themselves facing mortal illness. Thus, it is important to understand that these indicators are a guideline for treatment, not a crystal ball, and that you should not allow them to alter your determination to beat your lymphoma (Tables 6 and 7).

Table 6 IPI prognostic factors

- Age older than 60 years
- Eastern Cooperative Oncology Group performance score of 2 or more
- Elevated lactate dehydrogenase
- More than one site of extranodal involvement
- Stage III or stage IV lymphoma

Table 7 IPI risk categories

Risk category	IPI risk factors
Low	0 or 1
Low–intermediate	2
High–intermediate	3
High	4 or 5

28. Are all types of lymphoma treated the same way?

No. Because there are many different types of lymphoma, the approach to treatment depends on whether the goal is cure or disease control. Even if the lymphoma is considered incurable, many different treatments are available that can control the lymphoma, often for very long periods of time. These treatments, given intermittently, can be very effective for disease control, keeping lymphoma patients feeling well, often for many years. Especially in recent years, a large number of newer treatments have become available for lymphoma patients, and the outlook continues to improve at a rapid rate.

Newer techniques are becoming available to better distinguish between types of lymphoma that appear to be similar. Two patients may have a lymphoma that appears to be similar, yet with the same treatment, they may respond quite differently. At least some of the explanation for this lies in differences in which proteins are being produced by the lymphoma cells. Certain proteins may cause a lymphoma to grow more rapidly or be resistant to a particular treatment. These proteins are determined by genes that can be turned on or off in lymphoma cells. Analyzing these genes can help to better determine the features of the lymphoma and, it is hoped, to choose better treatments on the basis of this information. Gene chip technology is the method used to evaluate which genes, and therefore which proteins, are turned on in lymphoma cells. It is currently a research technique, but many studies are clearly demonstrating its importance in the management of lymphoma. It will be very important in the near future for helping to choose the correct treatment for different patients who appear to have the same type of lymphoma.

29. What types of treatment are available for lymphoma?

The options available for the management of lymphoma include observation, monoclonal antibody therapy, radioimmunotherapy, and chemotherapy with a number of different classes of drugs that have differing mechanisms of action and can be given either orally or by the intravenous route. External beam radiation can also be very useful in certain situations. Combinations of these different options are often administered together.

Chemotherapy refers to the use of drugs, usually given by mouth or in a vein (intravenously). After administration, the chemotherapy enters the bloodstream and travels to every part of the body. It can be given as either one drug alone (single-agent chemotherapy) or combined with other chemotherapy drugs (combination chemotherapy). A perfect chemotherapy drug would damage only cancer cells, but most drugs in use today can also damage normal cells, resulting in side effects. Chemotherapy can also be given in very high doses, having a greater effect against the lymphoma, but the side effect of this is destruction of the bone marrow. Giving high-dose chemotherapy along with the infusion of bone marrow stem cells is the basis for bone marrow or stem cell transplantation (discussed in Question 57). Radiation, another type of treatment, is usually given to specific areas of the body affected by lymphoma in order to control disease at that location. Sometimes it is administered to areas more prominently affected by the lymphoma after the administration of chemotherapy that was given to control more generalized disease. In this situation, it is used in an attempt to prevent the lymphoma from coming back at a particular site after treatment with chemotherapy.

30. How is indolent lymphoma treated?

After diagnosis and staging, the next step is to make decisions about treatment. As strange as it may seem, one of the options is something called "watch and wait." Other options include low doses of chemotherapy pills, more intensive intravenous chemotherapy, of which there is a growing list of options, **antibody therapy**, and transplant options. All of these options may be acceptable depending on the specific features of an individual patient's lymphoma, what treatment has previously been administered, and also the patient's personal preferences. You can discuss the merits of each of these approaches with your lymphoma doctor.

Antibody therapy
the use of antibodies to treat cancer.

The watch-and-wait concept has been around for many years and arose from observations that the indolent lymphomas often are slow growing, that frequently they are not associated with any symptoms, and that they can generally be controlled with therapy when it is necessary to prevent the lymphoma from causing problems. Earlier treatment has not yet been shown to prolong survival. Furthermore, as some treatments can have long-term harmful effects, saving their use for later when they may be more necessary helps to minimize this. Also, accepting watch and wait carries with it the understanding that the indolent lymphomas are not curable. Additional reasons to consider the watch-and-wait approach are the possible side effects from chemotherapy and also that the chemotherapy drugs work best the first time they are used. Therefore, keeping the drugs in reserve until symptoms or problems occur or seem likely to occur may be a valid strategy. Not every patient is comfortable with this approach, and indeed, some physicians feel that this is a defeatist attitude. Certainly, if you feel uncomfortable with this approach, you should discuss your feelings with your physician or obtain a second opinion. If symptoms are present or if the lymph node enlargement is causing problems, treatment will be recommended.

When watch and wait is acceptable, you should be seen on a regular basis by your lymphoma specialist. You should be alert for any symptoms that could indicate progression of lymphoma. Blood counts should be checked regularly, because any fall in the blood counts could signal disease progression. Occasionally, patients may go for many years without requiring treatment. Most patients, however, need some form of treatment after a few months to 2 years. For many patients and also some doctors, the idea of watch and wait is objectionable. Patients often prefer to be proactive and to feel in control as much as possible. These are valid reasons to choose treatment over watch and wait for some patients. Some of the arguments used to support watch and wait may not apply to the newer treatment options that have become available over the past few years. Whether earlier treatment with such agents can improve survival remains to be demonstrated in clinical trials.

If the decision is made to proceed with treatment, many options are available (shown in Table 8).

Table 8 Options available for the treatment of indolent lymphoma

Watch and wait
Chemotherapy pills
Intravenous chemotherapy in combination
Localized radiation (rarely)
Monoclonal antibody therapy
Radioimmunotherapy
Autologous stem cell transplant
Allogeneic stem cell transplant

Traditionally, chemotherapy is the first treatment that most patients with indolent lymphoma receive. More recently anti-CD20 monoclonal antibodies have become another treatment option. The challenge is to select the right agent or combination of agents best suited to the patient's circumstances. As noted previously, the approach to treating indolent lymphoma differs among physicians, but it is very important to discuss your physician's choice with him or her. Another option is to start with a milder chemotherapy regimen and to add the more aggressive chemotherapy for the later treatments. The rationale for this staged approach is to use less chemotherapy early, when the lymphoma is the most responsive to chemotherapy. Over time, the lymphoma is likely to be more resistant to chemotherapy, and stronger regimens will be needed. Giving stronger chemotherapy earlier has not been shown to prolong survival over milder chemotherapy and may add additional side effects that may cause more serious problems in later years or may interfere with quality of life.

On the other hand, many physicians feel that a more intensive treatment, although more likely to cause side effects, will produce a longer remission. This may allow patients to go longer before needing another type of treatment. One downside of this is that it is unlikely that, after receiving the more intensive treatments, the patients will subsequently respond to less intensive treatments. Certain patients will benefit from the less intensive treatments, often for many years, and the IPI or other measures may in the future allow such patients to be identified, thereby sparing them from the premature introduction of overly aggressive treatments. The aggressive combination chemotherapy regimens should generally be reserved for patients with indolent lymphoma with a more aggressive presentation or for patients who progress after treatment with less intensive treatments.

Nucleoside analogues are another group of agents that may be useful if you have indolent lymphoma. They are often used for the progression of the lymphoma occurring after treatment with aggressive chemotherapy or if the anthracycline containing chemotherapy is not used because of its effect on heart function; the nucleoside analogues may thus be a good choice for these patients. Because they can depress the immune system, you need to be especially watchful for any signs of infection. Because of its effect on the bone marrow, it can be more difficult to collect bone marrow stem cells for an autologous transplant after treatment with nucleoside analogues.

Among newer treatments for indolent lymphoma are the radio-immunotherapy agents, which have been developed from non-radioactive monoclonal antibodies. They have a radioactive molecule attached to the antibody. As a result, the radioactivity is carried directly to the lymphoma. The availability of these antibody treatments has dramatically changed the way that many types of lymphoma are treated.

High-dose therapy refers to the administration of very intensive chemotherapy with or without radiation. Because these high doses that are designed to maximally reduce the lymphoma also destroy the patient's own bone marrow, they are given in conjunction with an **autologous stem cell transplant** (discussed in Questions 59–61). The higher treatment doses may result in a longer remission in certain patients, but, unfortunately, this strategy does not offer a cure for indolent lymphoma.

Autologous stem cell transplant

a transplant in which one is one's own bone marrow stem cell donor.

An allogeneic transplant offers a different approach against lymphoma. This is the only treatment option that can potentially cure indolent lymphoma. This treatment uses bone marrow stem cells from a brother or sister or sometimes from an unrelated individual. Because there are significant risks associated with an allogeneic transplant, it is not a suitable treatment option for most patients with indolent lymphoma. This approach is discussed further in Question 58.

An allogeneic transplant offers a different approach against lymphoma. This is the only treatment option that can potentially cure indolent lymphoma.

Radiation therapy can be another useful option for the treatment of indolent lymphoma. Occasionally, patients may have stage I or II disease with one or two lymph node areas involved. In such cases, especially in the rare situation of stage I indolent lymphoma,

Radiation therapy

treatment using radiation.

radiation may actually provide a cure. If not a cure, it may actually delay the lymphoma from returning for many years.

31. How does my doctor know what treatment to recommend for my indolent lymphoma?

Your lymphoma specialist will make a recommendation for treatment after reviewing all aspects of your particular lymphoma and your general state of health and your own preferences after you have an understanding of the various options available. Consideration of your general health and well-being is important in determining your ability to tolerate the different chemotherapy drugs or combination regimens and the optimal time for therapy to begin. Your doctor's experience in treating other patients with similar types of lymphoma, knowledge gained from reading the medical literature, continuing medical education (attending lectures or conferences), and discussions with colleagues all provide the background for making treatment recommendations. Many centers, especially the larger cancer centers, have a number of lymphoma specialists who discuss all of the new cases of lymphoma at a regular conference. Discussions from these meetings can be very helpful when deciding on a treatment plan. Pathologists and radiologists will often also be at this meeting; thus, all aspects of the case can be considered together. The discussion can also serve to provide you with a number of second opinions. There are also a number of online resources available to physicians with up-to-date treatment recommendations. Medical journal reviews are also very helpful.

It can be quite frustrating when your physician presents a number of different treatment options and asks you to decide which treatment to receive. Given that many options may be right, you may need assistance in this decision; thus, you should ask your doctor for further guidance in making the best decision. Given a number of treatment options with similar outcomes, understanding the pros and cons of each one will be helpful to allow you to come to a decision on which one is right for you.

32. How is aggressive lymphoma treated?

The aggressive lymphomas are frequently fast growing and require treatment soon after the diagnosis is made. Because many patients can be cured, the approach involves giving the treatment that is the most likely to result in a cure as the initial therapy. After the diagnosis and staging have been completed, most patients receive six to eight cycles of chemotherapy.

For people whose lymphoma involves fewer lymph node areas (stage I or II), fewer cycles of therapy can safely be given. Studies have demonstrated that three cycles of chemotherapy followed by radiation are equivalent to six to eight cycles of chemotherapy in stage I or stage II aggressive (diffuse large B cell) lymphoma. Patients are therefore exposed to less chemotherapy, and the entire treatment course is shorter, potentially resulting in fewer complications from the treatment. Whether you can receive radiation and therefore be spared the extra cycles of chemotherapy depends on where the lymphoma is in your body. In some cases, it may be too risky to radiate particular areas of the body, and your doctor may prefer to administer six to eight cycles of chemotherapy.

Some patients, even though they receive six to eight cycles of chemotherapy, may still need radiation, especially if the site of lymphoma is bulky. Radiation to bulky sites that were present before chemotherapy, even if they have disappeared with treatment, may help prevent the lymphoma from returning at that site.

33. Is aggressive lymphoma curable if it returns after therapy or did not respond to therapy?

If your lymphoma either returns after chemotherapy or did not completely respond to therapy, a realistic chance of cure is still possible. High-dose chemotherapy with an autologous stem cell transplant is the most accepted treatment for people in otherwise good general health. In order to determine whether patients are likely to respond to the high-dose chemotherapy and transplant, another chemotherapy regimen is first given to shrink the lymphoma. If the lymphoma responds to this treatment, it is likely that a transplant is indicated. At this point, it is a good idea for you to be referred to a transplant center, where a transplant physician can determine whether you are likely to derive benefit from the transplant; if so, a number of tests to evaluate your heart, kidney, and lung functions and your general ability to withstand the transplant will be required. These tests should be performed as you are receiving your chemotherapy so that there is no delay between the chemotherapy and proceeding to the transplant. Of all patients who respond to the salvage chemotherapy and go on to receive an autologous transplant, approximately 35–40% will be cured. Many others may receive a benefit in terms of a longer period before the lymphoma returns. The chances of cure without a transplant in this setting are much smaller.

34. How is high-grade lymphoma treated?

In many cases, the very aggressive lymphomas can also be treated with either chemotherapy alone or combined with monoclonal antibody therapy. These are generally very rapidly growing lymphomas, frequently resulting in the development of often bulky lymph nodes in a short period of time with the potential to cause obstruction of vital structures including the airway or nerve tissue, with the potential for paralysis. As a result, treatment is generally fairly urgent. The treatment regimens used for these lymphomas consist of a number of different chemotherapy drugs given at frequent intervals. Patients usually require hospitalization for the few days each month when the chemotherapy is administered. These regimens are similar to the treatments used for childhood leukemia. Because most of these lymphomas are very fast growing, they can also be very sensitive to the effects of chemotherapy; therefore, there is a very high rate of complete response. As a result of the often very rapid response, the lymph nodes can shrink very fast, often over a period of days. As the cancer cells die, they release a lot of different toxic substances into the bloodstream, which then have to be safely excreted from the body. The kidneys need to be functioning well to handle the extra workload, and extra measures need to be taken in preparation for the chemotherapy in an attempt to prevent serious problems, including kidney failure. Intravenous fluids are given in large quanti-

In many cases, the very aggressive lymphomas can also be treated with either chemotherapy alone or combined with a monoclonal antibody.

ties, and the medication allopurinol is given to help the kidneys cope. A medication called rasburicase, which breaks down uric acid and sodium bicarbonate, may also be given to prevent these effects (called tumor lysis syndrome) from developing, but even with all of these measures, it still sometimes occurs.

Once a remission is achieved, further therapy is given to prevent the lymphoma from returning. More cycles of the same or similar chemotherapy may be given. The number of cycles varies, as there are a number of different regimens available. If the lymphoma is a B cell type and expresses **CD20** on the surface of the lymphoma cells, a monoclonal antibody directed against CD20 is also given along with the chemotherapy.

CD20

a protein on the surface of B lymphocytes and most B cell lymphomas.

An important aspect to treating high-grade lymphoma is treatment of the central nervous system if involved or to prevent reoccurrence of lymphoma at that site, which may occur even if there is no involvement at the time of diagnosis. This type of lymphoma has a higher possibility of central nervous system involvement than most other types. In order to evaluate the central nervous system, a **spinal tap** (lumbar puncture) is performed. The **spinal fluid** is analyzed for any lymphoma cells, and often, at the same time, a small amount of **intrathecal** chemotherapy is given through the spinal needle into the spinal fluid. The chemotherapy then circulates through the spinal fluid and the fluid around the brain. Giving this dose of chemotherapy before knowing whether the lymphoma involves the central nervous system does no harm. If there is central nervous system lymphoma, more intrathecal chemotherapy and possibly radiation will be necessary. Even if there is no lymphoma present in the spinal fluid, most patients with very

Spinal tap

the procedure for obtaining a sample of spinal fluid.

Spinal fluid

the fluid surrounding the brain and spinal cord.

Intrathecal

an injection into the fluid surrounding the spinal cord or brain.

aggressive lymphoma also need further intrathecal chemotherapy to prevent lymphoma from occurring at this site.

In some patients, especially if the lymphoma recurs during or after a complete treatment course, an autologous stem cell transplant with high-dose chemotherapy may be considered and can result in a cure.

PART FOUR

Chemotherapy and Radiation Therapy

What is chemotherapy?

What chemotherapy drug classes are used to treat lymphoma?

How is chemotherapy given?

More . . .

35. What is chemotherapy?

Paul Erlich (1854–1915) introduced the concept of chemotherapy. His revolutionary idea was to use mice to test antibiotics for activity against infectious disease. Subsequently, mice with tumors were used to test the activity of other chemicals against cancer. Further advances in the development of chemotherapy were made during World War I. Mustard gas was being tested as a chemical weapon, and exposure to this agent led to shrinkage of lymph nodes and bone marrow. These observations led to the use of nitrogen mustard for the treatment of lymphoma in the early 1940s.

"Chemotherapy" actually means the treatment of disease with any drug. However, in common usage, it refers to the treatment of cancer using drugs. Chemotherapy drugs are the most widely used treatments for lymphoma. Many different types of chemotherapy drugs are available, and new ones are continuously being developed. Many are derived from natural products found in the environment. The National Cancer Institute has a specific program in which scientists all over the world obtain samples from plants, trees, ocean-dwelling creatures, and so forth, and test them in the laboratory for any activity against cancer.

Intramuscular
an injection into the muscle.

Subcutaneous
underneath the skin.

Systemic treatment
a treatment, such as chemotherapy, that reaches all body parts through the bloodstream.

Local treatment
treatment aimed at a particular area of the body. For example, radiation treatment is local, whereas chemotherapy is systemic.

Chemotherapy drugs are given either orally or intravenously, or, less commonly, are injected directly into a muscle (**intramuscular**), under the skin (**subcutaneous**), or into the spinal fluid surrounding the brain and spinal cord (intrathecal). However the drugs are given, apart from intrathecally, the chemotherapy gets into the bloodstream and is distributed to all parts of the body. This type of treatment is referred to as **systemic treatment** and is different from **local treatment**, in which a specific site is targeted. Examples of local treatment include radiation and surgery. The benefit of chemotherapy over surgery or radiation is its ability to reach all parts of the lymphatic system. Depending on the specific type of lymphoma, even if lymph nodes in other areas are not enlarged, they may still be affected at the microscopic level and, therefore, benefit from chemotherapy. Surgery or radiation will not be helpful against these areas of microscopic involvement. Most chemotherapy drugs kill the more rapidly dividing cells. Lymphoma cells divide more rapidly than normal cells, especially the intermediate- and high-grade lymphomas. This explains their better response to chemotherapy than the indolent lymphomas. It also explains why chemotherapy affects the bone marrow, the lining of the gut, and eggs and sperm more than slower dividing cells.

Chemotherapy drugs are classified into groups based on their exact mechanism of action on cell machinery. Different groups of drugs act at different phases of the cell life cycle. Drugs acting on different mechanisms within cancer cells are often used together as combination chemotherapy regimens, having a greater effect against the cancer than single drugs.

36. What chemotherapy drug classes are used to treat lymphoma?

Many chemotherapy drugs are used to treat lymphoma. The number of available agents has increased, especially in the past few years. Drugs such as monoclonal antibodies are available and have the potential to increase the activity of chemotherapy drugs against lymphoma. Clinical studies continue to demonstrate better ways to use and combine the chemotherapy drugs that have been available for many years. Chemotherapy drugs can be used either alone or in combination, and they are usually given orally as pills or intravenously. When given intravenously, they can be given as a **bolus** (a quick injection), a short infusion, or a continuous infusion.

Bolus

a rapid intravenous injection.

Alkylating agents

a class of chemotherapy drugs.

Aplasia

a condition where blood cells are not produced.

There is one class of chemotherapy drugs called **alkylating agents**, which were the first chemotherapy drugs demonstrated to have anticancer activity in humans. During World War I, sulfur mustard gas was used as a weapon and was noted to produce **aplasia**, or shrinkage of lymph tissue. Subsequently, the related nitrogen mustards, which lacked the gases' nasty effects on the lungs and the skin, were examined for activity against lymphoma. Nitrogen mustard was developed as a result of such studies. Subsequently, other less toxic but more effective alkylating agents have been introduced. Alkylating agents cause cross-linking of DNA, adding an extra chemical group to the DNA strands. This prevents the cell from dividing, which is necessary for its normal growth. Without the ability to divide, the cell dies.

An important consideration when taking alkylating agents is the risk of second cancers. The risk for developing leukemia is estimated at approximately 6% and emphasizes the need to consider possible long-term complications of any treatment, especially for somebody without symptoms.

Antitumor antibiotics

a class of chemotherapy drugs.

Another chemotherapy drug class commonly used for the treatment of lymphoma belongs to a class of drugs called the **antitumor antibiotics**. They also cause cancer cells to die by interfering with the DNA.

Nucleoside analogues are another important group of drugs used in the treatment of lymphoma. They are taken up into lymphocytes and block the activity of an enzyme important for lymphocyte growth and are quite active against cells that divide only slowly, including the indolent lymphomas.

Nucleoside analogues
a type of chemotherapy drug that targets lymphocytes.

They are usually given by IV infusion for a variable number of cycles, depending on how well the patient responds. Some nausea or vomiting may occur but is unusual. Bone marrow suppression occurs, resulting in the need to monitor blood counts regularly. These drugs are also quite effective at killing normal lymphocytes, and this can be a very long-lasting effect. As a result, patients are at higher risk of developing certain infections such as **shingles** or even ***Pneumocystis carinii pneumoniae***, an infection more commonly seen in individuals with AIDS. Maintenance antibiotics can be very effective at preventing *Pneumocystis carinii pneumoniae* when given twice a week.

Shingles
a painful condition with a rash, usually affecting one area of the skin in the distribution of a nerve. It is due to reactivation of the chickenpox virus and usually occurs when the immune system is depressed.

Pneumocystis carinii pneumoniae
an infection affecting the lungs that can occur in people with an abnormal immune system.

Vinca alkaloids are another class of chemotherapy frequently used to treat lymphoma. The vinca alkaloids inhibit cancer cells by binding to **microtubules**, which prevent the cell from dividing normally. These drugs are given intravenously and usually are part of a combination chemotherapy regimen.

Vinca alkaloids
a type of chemotherapy drug.

Hair loss (**alopecia**) may occur with these drugs. The main side effect of vinca alkaloids is mild nerve damage. This is quite common, and the frequency increases with ongoing treatment. Often the first thing noticed is tingling in the fingers and toes. It is important at clinic visits to tell your physician about these changes. Jaw pain may also occur because the drug affects nerves in that area. Constipation as a result of this

Microtubules
structures present in individual cells that are important for allowing cells to divide.

Alopecia
hair loss.

class of chemotherapy affecting the nerves of the gut is also common, and, if necessary, you should take a stool softener or a laxative to prevent this complication. Nerve damage can occur and is generally reversible but may take many months to return to normal. Your doctor may reduce the dose or stop the drug completely, depending on your symptoms, which generally improve after the drug is discontinued.

There are several chemotherapy drugs and regimens available for treating lymphoma. Your physician should be happy to tell you about these drugs.

37. How is chemotherapy given?

Most patients with lymphoma receive chemotherapy intravenously. Other ways to administer the drugs include by mouth, under the skin, into the muscle, or into the cerebrospinal fluid (intrathecally).

If a number of cycles of chemotherapy are to be given intravenously, one very useful item is an **indwelling catheter**. Having a catheter can simplify the process of receiving chemotherapy infusions or injections. Indwelling catheters are essentially hollow tubes, one end of which is placed into a vein close to the heart. The other end of the tube is conveniently located under the skin or actually comes out through the skin, where it is available for connection to the chemotherapy bag. This prevents needing to find a vein and inserting a new intravenous needle each time that chemotherapy is given. It is also a safer way to administer chemotherapy. The catheters are also useful for taking blood samples. Blood transfusions, antibiotics, or intravenous fluids can also be given through the catheter.

Indwelling catheter

an intravenous catheter that can remain in place for longer than a few days.

Several different types of indwelling catheters exist and can remain in place for many months or even a year or more. Two main types of catheter exist and differ depending on whether it is entirely under the skin, as in the case of the **Portacath**, or if a part of it comes out through the skin (Figure 3).

The first type of catheter is a **Hickman** or **Broviac catheter**. Part of it is external, with approximately 6 inches of tubing outside the skin. This catheter requires dressing changes, and the tubes need to be flushed daily with a medication to keep blood from clotting in it. The patient can be taught to do this at home. The second type of catheter is a port or Portacath, which remains entirely under the skin without any external component. It does not require any dressing and requires only monthly flushing. The flushing requires the services of a nurse, and each time the port is accessed, it requires that a needle be inserted through the skin. In the case of both catheters, the part that is accessed for chemotherapy is usually placed on the upper part of the chest.

Portacath
an indwelling intravenous catheter that is placed entirely underneath the skin.

Hickman catheter
an intravenous line that passes through the skin into a large vein near the heart. It provides a safer and easier way to administer chemotherapy and obtain blood samples.

Broviac catheter
a type of catheter that goes directly into a large vein to allow easier administration of medications and blood tests.

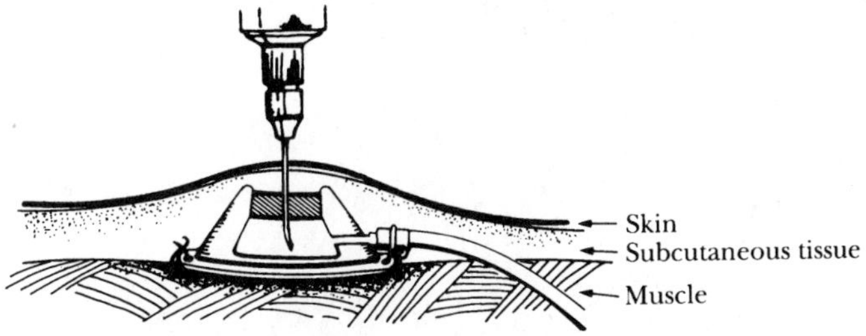

Figure 3 Schematic drawing of an implantable port. Reprinted from Yarbro CH, Frogge MH, Groenwald SL: *Cancer Nursing: Principles and Practice*, Sixth Ed. Copyright © 2000, Jones and Bartlett Publishers, LLC.

Smaller catheters may also be useful in some situations and may be placed in the arms instead of the chest wall, such as the percutaneous implantable central catheter or PICC (Figure 4).

38. What problems can result from having a catheter?

Interventional radiologist

a physician who is trained in using X-rays to aid in the performance of some types of surgical procedures.

Side effects from catheters do occur, but in most patients the convenience and comfort of a catheter outweigh its risks. A surgeon or an **interventional radiologist** (a doctor who performs surgical procedures such as placing an intravenous catheter using X-ray equipment) places these catheters, usually using local anesthesia. Complications rarely occur at the time that a catheter is first placed but include bleeding that is usually easily controlled. More seriously, but

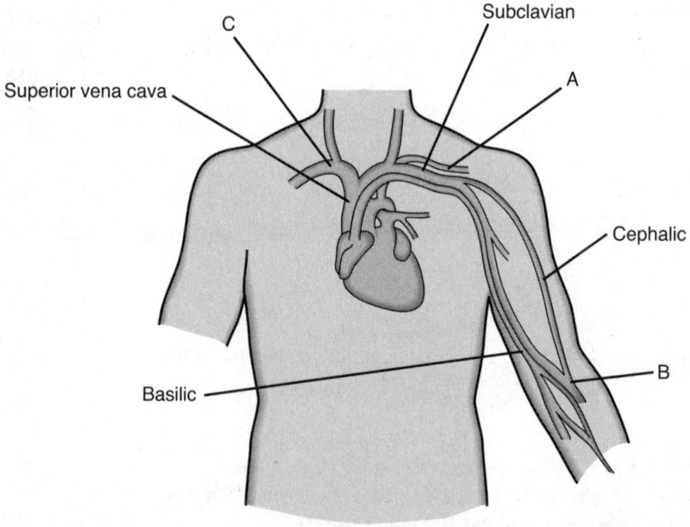

Figure 4 Sites of catheter placement: (A) percutaneous central venous catheters; (B) PICC lines; (C) can be in the subclavian vein on either side; the access for the catheter is usually placed in the upper chest wall and tunnelled under the skin to the point of insertion into the vein.

quite rarely, a lung can be punctured. Symptoms of a punctured lung include shortness of breath, cough, and chest pain. If there is any doubt, your doctor will obtain a chest X-ray.

Side effects from catheters do occur, but in most patients the convenience and comfort of a catheter outweigh its risks.

Complications that may develop during the time a catheter is in place can include infection or a blood clot forming around the catheter. Thus, some doctors place patients on a low dose of coumadin, a blood thinner, in an attempt to prevent blood clots.

If you want an indwelling catheter and your healthcare team recommends this approach, you can discuss which catheter is the most appropriate.

39. What are the side effects of chemotherapy?

In this question, we discuss general side effects that may occur with most chemotherapy drugs. The extent of side effects varies depending on the specific drugs that you receive, how they are administered, and how your body reacts to them. Your doctor and nurse will explain the side effects that you are most likely to experience. Most people associate nausea, vomiting, and hair loss with chemotherapy, but this is variable from person to person depending on the chemotherapy regimen. Today, good drugs are available to prevent nausea and vomiting. Thus, if you experience nausea or vomiting the first time that you receive chemotherapy, ask your physician whether any changes can be made for future treatments.

Most chemotherapy drugs kill some normal cells as well as lymphoma cells. Some of the side effects that you experience result from damage to these normal cells. The normal cells that are the most affected are those in areas where cells grow and divide most rapidly. These areas include hair follicles, bone marrow, the **gastrointestinal tract**, and the **reproductive system**. Thus, the most common side effects are hair loss, mouth sores, diarrhea, and problems related to infertility, although you should remember that having had chemotherapy does not necessarily mean that you are infertile. Because most chemotherapy drugs have severe effects on sperm and eggs, it is very important not to conceive while receiving chemotherapy. Appropriate contraception practices should be used if there is any potential for pregnancy.

Gastrointestinal tract

the gut, from mouth to anus.

Reproductive system

the body parts associated with reproduction.

40. Will I lose my hair?

Many patients undergoing chemotherapy are understandably anxious about hair loss. Your doctor and nurse will discuss the likelihood of this in your case. The likelihood of hair loss and how much to expect depends on the chemotherapy drugs that you receive, how frequently they are given, and the duration of treatment. For many patients, especially women, hair loss can be the most traumatic part of the entire treatment process. Loss of hair is a very obvious change in your appearance and can understandably have a considerable affect on self-esteem. It may be the most visible sign, especially among women, that there is a problem. It can occur in other areas apart from the scalp. A loss of facial hair (mustache and beard), axillary (underarm) hair, and pubic hair occurs with the longer chemotherapy regimens. The hair loss can vary, with some people experiencing thinning and others experiencing complete hair loss. The hair loss associated with chemotherapy usually begins 2 to 4 weeks after your treatment has begun. It is usually temporary and grows back starting 1 to 2 months after the completion of therapy. Your new hair may have a different texture or color; for example, it may grow back curly, whereas before chemotherapy it was straight.

The hair loss associated with chemotherapy usually begins 2 to 4 weeks after your treatment has begun. It is usually temporary and grows back starting 1 to 2 months after the completion of therapy.

How can I cope with hair loss?

First, discuss hair loss with your physician and nurse, your close family members, and/or your friends. You may wish to purchase a wig before your first treatment begins so that the color and texture can be closely matched to your own hair color. Many patients prefer to wear a head scarf or bandana rather than a wig, whereas others prefer no head covering. The best thing to do is whatever feels right to you. The American Cancer Society offers an entire program that addresses hair loss and how it affects your appearance. The program is called "Look Good, Feel Better," and it offers seminars as well as one-on-one appointments with professional hair stylists and makeup artists. It offers fashion tips for wearing scarves as well as wigs. Information about this program is available from the American Cancer Society through a toll-free number (1-800-395-LOOK) that operates 24 hours a day, 7 days a week. The American Cancer Society also offers wigs that are free of charge, and some insurance companies will cover the cost of wigs. Otherwise, the cost should be tax deductible.

41. Will I have nausea and vomiting with treatment?

Years ago, patients receiving chemotherapy may have gotten very sick and experienced much vomiting. Today, however, there are many more chemotherapy drugs and other treatments that do not cause significant nausea and/or vomiting. In addition, there are many antinausea (**antiemetic**) medications that are very effective in preventing this problem. If necessary, your physician will prescribe antinausea drugs along with your chemotherapy. If you are still having nausea or vomiting, inform your doctor or nurse so that they can alter your antinausea drug regimen. Do not assume that you have to tough it out. Also, because everybody responds differently to different regimens, the first antinausea regimen may not work well for you, and alternatives are available. Sometimes a small dose of a steroid can be beneficial when added to other antinausea medications.

Antiemetic
a medication to prevent nausea and vomiting.

Also, rather than eating regular-sized meals, eating several smaller meals throughout the day can be helpful. You should avoid fried or fatty foods and should eat and drink slowly. Although rest is also helpful after a meal, you should not lie flat for at least 2 hours after eating.

42. Do I need to change my diet?

Good nutrition, although frequently neglected in the American diet, is always important. The same applies, even more so, as you proceed in your fight against lymphoma. What good nutrition means will vary according to your specific circumstances. Consulting with a dietician can be helpful. Eating adequate amounts of a healthy diet can help you feel better in general. When your body is receiving all that it needs, your ability to tolerate the side effects of the lymphoma and its treatment is increased, and you may also decrease your chance of infection through a beneficial effect on the immune system. A healthy diet and good nutrition will enhance your ability to maintain your strength and energy level, counteracting fatigue.

For those of you who do not have any specific problems that interfere with your appetite or ability to eat, we suggest that you follow the guidelines set by the U.S. Department of Agriculture, which outline what to eat on a daily basis (www.choosemyplate.gov). Use this as a rough guide, possibly adding one to two servings from the dairy group and one to two servings from the protein foods group. This will increase your total protein intake, which often is needed during an illness.

Changing your diet is a relatively easy step to take and is an aspect of your health in which you can have direct control. This is important at a time when you may feel that so many things fall outside of your control. Making your diet healthier may carry the benefits discussed previously, but as far as we know will not directly treat the lymphoma. Even the National Cancer Institute's stance is that there is not any evidence that any specific kind of diet or food alone can either cure cancer or keep it from coming back.

If you have lost weight, you may be able to focus on increasing your protein and energy (caloric) intake. If your appetite is good, this is fairly easy to accomplish. Focus on eating more high-calorie foods that provide protein, such as milk, cheese, and eggs. Sauces and gravies are also an efficient way of obtaining more calories.

If your appetite is poor, the same high-calorie and high-protein diet is encouraged. Try to eat several (five or six) small meals throughout the day and to include high-protein snacks such as ice cream, pudding, cheese, and peanut butter. At those times when you are not able to face a meal, a nourishing drink is an acceptable alternative. You can also add these drinks between meals to help with weight gain. At certain times during chemotherapy, especially when your white blood cell count is low, you may be restricted to a **low microbial diet**—one that limits your exposure to food-borne bacteria or fungi.

Low microbial diet
a diet containing low amounts of bacteria or fungi.

Several different commercially available supplements can add calories and protein to your diet. These taste best when served very cold. If the taste of one brand or flavor does not appeal to you, try another. Many people doctor up these drinks; for example, if the chocolate variety is too chocolaty or too sweet, try mixing it in a blender with some milk or vanilla ice cream. Alternatively, try adding some fruit, milk, or other flavor of ice cream to a vanilla variety drink. You can also create a milk shake from scratch. Or, combine milk with various fruits or fruit yogurt to make a smoothie. You can also add a scoop of ice cream and a few teaspoons of protein powder. Although these powders are commonly available, you should consult your health-care team before using any dietary supplements.

At times you may want some foods that may be considered unhealthy. You may need to eat whatever food you can to obtain enough calories. Sometimes you may need to think of food like medicine: take some every 2 to 3 hours whether you feel like it or not. Be conscious of what you are eating, but, on the other hand, do not become obsessed. Mealtimes should be enjoyable and not a source of stress.

If you do not feel like preparing a meal, frozen dinners and microwaveable foods are convenient. This is also a perfect opportunity to give family and friends the chance to help you (e.g., going to the grocery store or doing some cooking). If you have times when your energy level is better and you enjoy cooking, you could prepare some meals in advance and freeze them for later. If you really cannot face preparing or eating a meal, have one of the nutritional supplements discussed previously.

Dehydration
low fluids in the body, which can cause dizziness, fatigue, fainting, and other minor symptoms. If not corrected, dehydration can cause more serious problems.

43. What should I do if I'm having side effects that interfere with eating?

A sore throat or mouth sores from chemotherapy or radiation can result in difficulty eating. Crunchy foods such as raw fruits and vegetables, dry breads and cereals, spicy foods, and citrus should be avoided. Instead, eat soft and creamy food such as yogurt, pudding, buttered noodles, and cooked cereal. You may also find that foods that are too hot can also cause discomfort. Lukewarm or cool foods tend to be more soothing.

If you cannot tolerate solids, try liquid foods such as cream soups or nutrition drinks and shakes.

If nausea or vomiting is a problem, try sipping fluids throughout the day (along with trying antinausea medications), because you need to drink enough fluids to prevent **dehydration**. Water is good, but juice-type commercial supplements may be even better. These provide protein as well as calories.

If nausea or vomiting is a problem, try sipping fluids throughout the day (along with trying antinausea medications), because you need to drink enough fluids to prevent dehydration.

If you're feeling queasy but are not vomiting, try eating bland foods that are easy to digest (e.g., crackers, toast, rice, gelatin, and sherbet). These foods are not adequate sources of protein, calories, or nutrients, but this diet can be followed for a few days until the nausea subsides, as long as you are drinking enough liquids.

Sometimes food that you have previously enjoyed may taste bland. This can be the result of various medications, including chemotherapy. This change in taste may result in a loss of appetite and a failure to obtain adequate nutrition. Again, treating food likc medicine—eating small amounts at regular intervals—may be a way to overcome this problem. You may need to experiment with new foods or new seasonings, or may need to add additional sugar, salt, or other flavor to enhance the taste. Most people report that cold or room-temperature foods are less offensive in their smell and taste.

Anorexia
loss of appetite.

Megestrol acetate
a medication that can increase the appetite.

If you simply have no appetite (**anorexia**), you may benefit from **megestrol acetate**, which is a hormonal agent that can stimulate the appetite and result in a weight gain. This is an option that you should discuss with your physician.

Hematocrit
a measure of the number of red cells, useful for anemia or polycythemia (too many red cells).

Palpitations
the sensation of an irregular heartbeat.

44. How do I cope with anemia?

Anemia is common in patients with lymphoma. A blood test measures the hemoglobin level, or the **hematocrit**. Symptoms of anemia include fatigue, weakness, shortness of breath, headache, ringing in your ears, **palpitations** (an increased awareness of the heart beating), nausea, and occasional chest pain.

Anemia can occur for many different reasons. Often, bone marrow reacts to lymphoma in your body by decreasing the production of red blood cells. This also happens in people with many other illnesses, not just cancer. It occurs with infections and arthritis. This type of anemia is called **anemia of chronic disease**.

Anemia of chronic disease
an anemia caused by the bone marrow's reaction to being sick.

Lymphoma involving the bone marrow can also cause anemia. Bleeding can obviously lead to anemia and also needs to be considered as a cause. If bleeding occurs, report it to your physician. Having black, tarry bowel movements is a sign of bleeding in the bowels and requires urgent attention.

Chemotherapy commonly causes or worsens anemia and may contribute to fatigue (Question 47). You should note that anemia is only one of many factors that contribute to fatigue.

Your doctor may perform tests to determine the reasons for the anemia. Deficiencies of iron, vitamin B_{12}, or folic acid are possible causes that simple blood tests can easily evaluate. If any of these are deficient, supplements can be provided. More commonly, anemia is not due to any deficiency in your diet and is therefore unlikely to respond to dietary supplements. Question 47 discusses the use of **erythropoietin** in preventing or treating anemia.

Erythropoietin
a hormone produced by the kidneys that stimulates the bone marrow to produce red blood cells.

When you have symptoms from anemia, you should not overdo activities. Exercising is generally a good thing and should be encouraged but not pushed too hard. Limiting your activities to what you feel up to and getting plenty of rest can help to improve your sense of well-being.

45. Why is having a low white blood count such a concern?

Neutropenia

a low level of neutrophils.

Another common effect of chemotherapy is the reduction of the white blood cell count (**neutropenia**), which increases the risk of developing an infection. Crowds and people with colds or flu should be avoided, but in reality, the most common infections during periods of a low blood count actually arise from within your own body. A neutropenic or low microbial diet may help to prevent some of these infections. The chance of an infection is increased for older patients or for those with other medical problems such as chronic lung disease or diabetes. Having a central venous catheter also increases the chance of an infection. Even if you take precautions, infections are not entirely preventable. The risk of infection is highest with lower white blood cell counts and is also related to longer durations of neutropenia. Certain chemotherapy drugs or combinations of drugs are associated with a higher risk of infections than others.

If a fever develops while you are receiving chemotherapy or in the period afterward when your white count is low, you should seek medical attention without delay, especially if it is above 100.5°F. With neutropenia, infections can progress very rapidly and can even result in death if antibiotics are not started promptly.

The development of a fever may result in a hospital admission. For this reason, it is a good idea to keep a weekend bag packed. Sometimes, after the fever is assessed, an outpatient antibiotic treatment may be adequate. First, blood samples should be obtained before starting antibiotics to identify the cause of the infection. You will also have a chest X-ray, and a urine culture will need to be examined.

Depending on the chemotherapy that you receive and on other factors such as your age and general health, your physician may prescribe a white blood cell growth factor in an effort to allow your white blood cell count to recover sooner after chemotherapy. Most commonly, granulocyte-colony stimulating factor, or G-CSF, is used for this purpose. It is administered by a daily subcutaneous injection until the white blood cell count has recovered. A chemically altered version of G-CSF is also available. It remains in the circulation for a considerably longer period of time until the white blood cell count recovers and therefore only needs to be given once with every chemotherapy cycle. The longer lasting version of the colony stimulating factor is also given as a subcutaneous injection.

Not everybody on chemotherapy needs to get a white blood cell growth factor. The decision is based on how likely you are to get an infection while on chemotherapy and whether you have previously experienced an infection. Discuss the need for a growth factor with your physician. The American Society of Clinical Oncology has developed guidelines for when these growth factors should be administered.

46. How do lymphoma and its treatment affect my sexuality?

It is not uncommon for lymphoma and its treatment to bring about physical and/or emotional changes that affect your sexual relationship. The degree to which this occurs depends on several factors, including the stage and symptoms of your lymphoma, the treatment that you are undergoing, as well as your overall emotional state.

It is difficult for some people to initiate conversations about sexuality with their partner; however, it can be very beneficial to speak openly and honestly with each other about your needs and wants. If you cannot do this, you might find it helpful to see a counselor or therapist on a short-term basis.

Although it may be even harder to discuss sexuality with strangers, a discussion with your healthcare team may help you to adjust to any changes as they occur. If your doctor or nurse is not helpful, speaking to the social worker may be beneficial.

One common issue that you may face as a result of your lymphoma and your treatment is a decreased sex drive, which can be a direct effect of your treatment or associated with fatigue or stress. It is important that this does not become the cause of further stress in your relationship. With good communication, your partner should understand the reasons for the decreased **libido**. You can also remind your partner that this is a temporary disruption, and once treatment (or the fatigue associated with it) is over, your sex drive will return to its former level. Depression, which is treatable, should also be considered as a possible cause for decreased libido.

Libido
sex drive.

Chemotherapy and radiation can cause dryness of a woman's vagina. A water-soluble lubricant can help ease discomfort associated with decreased vaginal lubrication. Also, keep an open mind that there are different ways to feel sexual pleasure, as there may be times when intercourse is not possible. It is very important that you and your partner continue other ways of expressing affection for each other. Sometimes just cuddling can be enough, or you may want to explore other ways of caressing and stimulating each other.

Chemotherapy and radiation can also result in low **testosterone** levels, which result in difficulty obtaining or maintaining an erection. Replacing testosterone may be all that is required. Sometimes antidepressants may interfere with a man's ability to function during intercourse.

Testosterone
a male hormone.

If your white blood cell or platelet count is low (50,000 is usually the minimum requirement), sexual intercourse may not be advisable; you should discuss this with your healthcare team. Lymphoma cannot be passed through sexual intercourse. However, small amounts of chemotherapy can be present in semen of men receiving treatment, so condoms are highly recommended.

Some people choose to wait to focus on the sexual part of their relationship until treatment is complete. Only you and your partner can decide what is best. Honesty and open communication avoid hurt feelings and misunderstandings and are an important part of resuming normal sexual activity.

47. Is fatigue always due to chemotherapy?

Fatigue, a very common symptom for many patients with cancer, can vary from slight fatigue, making everyday activities slightly more burdensome, to profound fatigue, resulting in extreme difficulty even getting out of bed. Fatigue can be extremely incapacitating, resulting in major impairment in quality of life, and is common even in patients who are not receiving chemotherapy. Many causes of fatigue exist among cancer patients, with anemia being one. This may be related to lymphoma's bone marrow involvement, resulting in decreased red blood cell production. Even without bone marrow involvement, anemia of chronic disease may also be present and may contribute to fatigue, which cytokine production can cause. Cytokines are chemicals that tumor cells produce in response to an infection. Lymphoma patients are understandably under a lot of stress, which is another cause of fatigue. Depression can add to the fatigue. Medications should also be evaluated as an additional factor that contributes to stress.

Discuss fatigue with your physician or nurse if it is an issue. If anemia is a significant component causing fatigue, a blood transfusion may be necessary. Erythropoietin is a hormone that stimulates red blood cell production. Apart from being produced in the body, it is also available for injection and may be beneficial in some circumstances (the kidneys produce erythropoietin, which then travels to the bone marrow cells and stimulates the production of red blood cells). It is available as a medication in a number of different preparations, which are given by a subcutaneous or intravenous injection, has been used for many years and is very similar to the naturally produced erythropoietin that the kidneys produce. The injections can be given either three times per week or once per week. There is a longer-acting version that can be given every 2 weeks and appears to be similarly effective to the injections given more frequently. Because there are many other causes of fatigue besides anemia, erythropoietin will not benefit all patients. Discuss this with your physician. Your list of medications should also be evaluated. If any medications can be discontinued, this may be helpful. Again, discuss this with your physician.

Maintaining a good caloric intake and adequate hydration is also important in counteracting fatigue. Plan your daily activities with an emphasis on the activities that are more important. It is quite acceptable to take naps, but sleeping too much during the day can further disrupt your sleeping pattern. Some daily exercise as tolerated can also be helpful in managing your fatigue.

48. Does chemotherapy cause bleeding?

Chemotherapy may cause bleeding, which is due to a fall in the platelet count. Regular blood counts are important while you are receiving chemotherapy and will help to detect the need for platelet transfusions. If you develop any abnormal bleeding while on chemotherapy, inform your doctor. Abnormal bruising in addition to bleeding is also important. Other signs of a low platelet count include **petechiae**, which are small, purple, reddish spots on your skin that are actually tiny bleeds. They are most frequently seen on the front of your shins. During periods when your platelet count is low, you should avoid razor blades for shaving (use electric razors instead), nail clippers, and dental floss.

Petechiae

pinpoint red spots that occur with low platelet counts and are due to tiny areas of bleeding into the skin.

For mouth care, you should use only a very soft toothbrush or sponges.

The occurrence of low platelet counts during chemotherapy depends on a number of factors, including the type of chemotherapy being administered, the amount of chemotherapy that the patient has previously received, and whether and to what degree the bone marrow is involved with lymphoma. It is important to control high blood pressure when the platelet count is low, as the risk of bleeding may be increased.

Activities such as contact sports that could result in trauma need to be curtailed while the platelet count is low. Discuss any such activities with your physician before participation.

49. What is radiation therapy?

Radiation therapy uses high-energy x-rays to kill or prevent cancer cells from growing.

Simulation

the planning necessary before administering any radiation treatment.

Radiation therapy uses high-energy X-rays to kill or prevent cancer cells from growing. Cancer cells grow faster than normal cells, so they are more susceptible to radiation. Because radiation therapy can also damage normal tissues around the area being radiated, your radiation doctor will try to ensure that only the cancer cells receive the radiation. Before starting radiation treatment, a **simulation** will be performed, at which time tiny tattoo marks or dots will be placed on your skin to mark the area to be radiated. Areas that are not to receive radiation will be protected with lead shielding. The radiation treatment itself takes only a few minutes, but treatment is spread over a few days to a few weeks, depending on the total dose of radiation to be administered. For treatment, you will generally be lying on a table close to a noisy radiation machine.

Before starting radiation treatment, you will have an appointment with a radiation oncologist, who specializes in radiation therapy to treat cancer. At the initial visit, your case will be reviewed to ensure that you are to benefit from radiation treatment and that the treatment can be given safely. The radiation oncologist will also review any scans or X-ray tests, as these will be helpful for planning the exact area that needs radiation. After this visit, you should have a good understanding of the reasons for needing radiation treatment, what to expect from the radiation in terms of side effects, and how long the treatment course will be.

Radiation is referred to as local treatment, being useful when treating particular sites within the body. The field of treatment is called a radiation port. **Total body irradiation** refers to the radiation of the whole body and is sometimes used in preparation for a bone marrow transplant.

Total body irradiation
radiation therapy administered to the entire body, usually in preparation for a transplant.

50. Will I need radiation therapy?

Radiation therapy can be useful for the treatment of lymphoma under many different circumstances. It can be used as the only treatment for some patients depending on the type and stage of lymphoma. Therefore, accurate staging is very important for planning the correct treatment.

For patients with aggressive non-Hodgkin's lymphoma, radiation, if needed, is usually combined with chemotherapy. In fact, in certain situations, using radiation therapy allows the number of chemotherapy cycles necessary to be reduced, therefore reducing the risk of side effects from chemotherapy exposure. In other situations, the radiation may be an additional treatment aimed at areas where the lymphoma was particularly bulky, in an attempt to reduce the likelihood of recurrence.

Radiation can rapidly control lymphoma at specific sites if necessary. An example of such a need is pain control due to lymphoma growing at one site or lymphoma pressing on the spinal cord, causing nerve damage. Spinal cord compression is a very urgent situation in which the lymphoma presses on the spinal cord, causing weakness (often in the legs), numbness, and possible loss of control of bladder or bowel function. These symptoms require extremely urgent medical attention, because unless they are corrected rapidly, the nerve damage may be permanent.

51. What are the side effects of radiation therapy?

Radiation therapy itself is painless and does not cause you to become radioactive; however, you may experience some side effects depending on the part of your body that is being radiated. Other factors include the dose of radiation and whether chemotherapy is given at the same time. Side effects may be localized to the body part being treated or can be more widespread. Be sure to report any and all side effects to your healthcare team, as most can be effectively managed. Also remember that although side effects can be unpleasant, most are temporary and will gradually disappear after the treatment is finished.

During radiation therapy, the skin in the area being treated may become dry, irritated, and sensitive; it may feel and look sunburned and may also become itchy and then peel. To avoid further irritation, radiated areas should be kept clean using only warm water and very mild cleansers. Your healthcare team may prescribe or recommend creams, lotions, or ointments. You should avoid all cosmetics, deodorants, perfumes, powders, and other products that increase irritation in the affected area and that your healthcare team has not approved. It is also important to avoid sun exposure for a long time after therapy has been completed.

Radiation may also cause hair loss to the specific body part being treated. Although this is generally temporary, higher doses can also cause permanency. Unlike chemotherapy, radiation treatment does not cause generalized hair loss.

Fatigue, or generalized weakness, is another common side effect of radiation therapy. It tends to increase gradually and is cumulative as radiation continues.

Fatigue, or generalized weakness, is another common side effect of radiation therapy. It tends to increase gradually and is cumulative as radiation continues. By completion of a course of radiation therapy, many patients have a significant degree of fatigue.

Medical problems—including infection, anemia, and dehydration, all of which are treatable—can compound fatigue that is caused by radiation. Your physician should look for any of these aggravating factors. Ways of coping with fatigue include ensuring adequate sleep at night, resting during the day, eating a balanced diet with adequate calories and protein, and exercising at a tolerable level. Light exercise, such as walking and stretching, is helpful. A consultation with a physical therapist may prove helpful for advice on incorporating light exercise into your daily routine.

Radiation can cause a loss of appetite (anorexia) or nausea (Questions 41 and 43). Radiation treatments to the neck or chest may result in a sore throat or dry mouth, resulting in a condition called **xerostomia**, which results from damage to the salivary glands. Saliva is essential for chewing and swallowing food and is the primary lubricant for food. Inflammation to the **esophagus** (the tube that connects the throat to your stomach) may also occur. This condition, called **esophagitis**, results in painful or difficult swallowing and possibly also heartburn.

Xerostomia

dryness of the mouth due to disease.

Esophagus

the tube connecting the throat to the stomach.

Esophagitis

inflammation of the esophagus.

If you experience esophagitis or xerostomia, consider eating softer foods or commercially available dietary shakes. You should avoid citrus fruits and juices, as these can be especially irritating. Commercially available saliva substitutes may also be helpful for coping with a dry mouth; your healthcare team can help with this.

PART FIVE

Other Therapies

What is immunotherapy?

What are monoclonal antibodies?

How are monoclonal antibodies administered?

More . . .

52. What is immunotherapy?

Immunotherapy

treatment aimed at controlling the immune system.

Biologic therapy

treatment that focuses the body's immune system on diseased cells.

Immunotherapy, sometimes referred to as **biologic therapy**, is a treatment that involves the use of the immune system to treat the disease. These treatments include monoclonal antibodies, radioimmunotherapies, therapeutic vaccines, as well as allogeneic stem cell transplants.

53. What are monoclonal antibodies?

Monoclonal antibodies are immunoglobulin proteins that are produced by one population of cells or clone (hence monoclonal). Every antibody is built in the shape of the letter "Y." This structure allows the antibody to be useful for fighting infection. It also makes it useful for treating some types of cancer. The arms of the "Y" have a particular protein sequence that can recognize and attach to small, specific protein targets, termed "antigens". The foot of the "Y" can link to other cells in the immune system that can rid the body of the antigen. Antibodies are vital to a normal immune system, providing essential protection against otherwise potentially fatal infections.

Another way to help understand monoclonal antibodies is to know that we all have white blood cells that are specialized in making antibodies. These plasma cells are the most mature B cell in our immune system. Each plasma cell is responsible for one type of antibody. In turn, each antibody acts specifically against one specific antigen. Antigens are proteins located on the surface of all cells, which our immune system uses to determine whether cells are a necessary part of the body or need to be destroyed. Lymphoma treatments now available consist of large amounts of antibodies that can be specifically directed to a single antigen on a cell's surface. An analogy often used is that the monoclonal antibody is a guided missile that hones in on lymphoma cells and destroys them.

CD20 is an antigen that is present on the lymphoma cells of most patients who have indolent non-Hodgkin's lymphoma. Anti-CD20 antibodies are designed so that the arms of the "Y" attach to CD20. When this antibody is infused into the circulation, it seeks out the CD20 that is present on lymphocytes and targets them for destruction.

54. How are monoclonal antibodies administered?

Monoclonal antibodies used to treat lymphoma are infused intravenously according to varying schedules. If given along with chemotherapy, the schedule depends on the chemotherapy regimen.

The first time a monoclonal antibody is infused, patients are likely to experience fever and chills, which can be quite uncomfortable, but this resolves by slowing the infusion. These symptoms generally decrease with subsequent infusions, but if the reaction is severe the infusion should be stopped.

Because of this, the first infusion takes the longest, maybe even more than 8 hours. Subsequent infusions can generally be completed in shorter times. These symptoms generally decrease with subsequent infusions. Fever and chills occur less often with the remaining infusions. Acetaminophen and diphenhydramine can help to reduce the severity of the fever and chills.

55. How is radioimmunotherapy administered?

Nuclear medicine

the medicine specialty that deals with using radioisotopes for obtaining body scans and for treatment.

These antibodies are more complicated to administer than non-radioactive monoclonal antibodies. Because they are a form of radiation treatment, a **nuclear medicine** physician or a radiation oncologist is required for its administration. Only one course of treatment is necessary, but it takes 7 to 9 days. The first administration on day 1 takes a number of hours. Next, a modified form of radioactive antibody is administered to give a determination of the amount of radiation that different parts of the body will receive when the radioactive antibody is administered. Because of the need for special handling of radiation treatments, it may be necessary to receive the two treatments in different locations, which can be inconvenient.

Gamma camera

a nuclear imaging camera that can detect radioactivity.

Within 1 or 2 days, a scan is performed with a **gamma camera** in order to determine the distribution of the radiation in the body. Additional scans may be necessary 2 to 4 days later, depending on the results of the first scan.

It is currently recommended that radioactive antibodies be given only to patients whose platelet count is at least 100,000 as a further drop in blood counts may occur, sometimes resulting in the need for transfusions. A bone marrow examination is also recommended before this treatment. If more than 25% of the marrow space is involved with lymphoma, radioactive antibodies should not be given, as there is a risk that too much radiation will be concentrated in the marrow, possibly resulting in permanent marrow damage.

56. What are lymphoma vaccines?

You are familiar with vaccines given during childhood to prevent infections. A **vaccine** is a preparation of a protein given to stimulate an immune response against a particular infection. Vaccination for cancer is a newer concept. In lymphoma, vaccination is experimental.

Vaccine
a preparation of a protein given to stimulate an immune response against a particular infection.

The aim of treatment is to eliminate lymphoma or to prevent its reoccurrence. With immunization against an infectious disease, the aim is to prevent the infection from occurring in the first place.

For a vaccine to be effective in cancer, a protein unique to the cancer cell is needed to stimulate an immune response. For most cancers, this is not currently available, because their proteins also occur in normal cells.

In B cell lymphomas, the abnormal cells have a single type of immunoglobulin on their surface. This immunoglobulin is an antibody molecule, and part of it is called an **idiotype**. The idiotype is the same for all the lymphoma cells belonging to that patient but differs from the idiotype on other normal lymphocytes and also from the lymphoma of other patients. As a result, the idiotype is an excellent target for vaccination.

Idiotype
a protein sequence on the surface of B lymphocytes that is like a fingerprint. All related lymphocytes contain the same protein sequence.

The first step in producing a lymphoma vaccine is the surgical removal of a lymph node. The specific idiotype is then produced during a process that takes

8 to 16 weeks. Once produced, the idiotype is joined to another large foreign carrier protein that enhances the immune response, and the carrier protein is then ready for injection into the patient. The vaccination is given along with a growth factor. The vaccination schedule varies according to the particular clinical trial. To date, a number of clinical centers are conducting clinical trials to determine the best vaccination approach. Thus far, results appear promising, and much more information should become available in the near future.

57. What is a bone marrow or stem cell transplant?

A bone marrow or stem cell transplant is a treatment that allows for the administration of higher doses of chemotherapy or radiation than you could receive without the transplant. Currently, the effects on the bone marrow limit the ability to increase the dose of many drugs that are used to treat lymphoma. Being able to increase the dose of the drugs can reduce the chance that the lymphoma will return. In the case of some chemotherapy drugs, this increased dose could destroy the bone marrow. If such a case were to occur, a very high risk of infection is likely, and patients would require regular transfusions of both red blood cells and platelets. In order to avoid this complication, a bone marrow or stem cell transplant can be performed.

A bone marrow transplant, as the name suggests, involves actually using the bone marrow stem cells for the transplant. Obtaining the bone marrow requires an operation with a general anesthetic. This procedure is performed less commonly now, and most transplant centers obtain stem cells from the peripheral circulation rather than directly from the bone marrow. Such transplants are called **peripheral blood stem cell transplants**. Although obtained from the blood, the stem cells are still bone marrow stem cells, but they move into the bloodstream after treatment with growth factors such as G-CSF. Stem cells also move into the blood circulation as blood counts recover after chemotherapy. Often a patient's own stem cells are collected after the administration of both chemotherapy and white blood cell growth factors. When transplanted back into the patient after high-dose chemotherapy, the stem cells are able to produce red blood cells, white blood cells, and platelets. Using stem cells obtained from the blood as opposed to the marrow results in a significantly shorter period of low blood counts. This has enabled patients to have shorter hospital stays or possibly even to have such a treatment performed as an outpatient.

Peripheral blood stem cell transplant
a transplant using marrow stem cells that have been obtained from the blood circulation.

58. Why is a transplant used for treating lymphoma?

Basically, there are two main mechanisms by which a transplant can be useful in treating lymphoma. First, it enables the safer delivery of much higher doses of chemotherapy than would otherwise be possible. The higher doses of chemotherapy may cure an aggressive lymphoma or prevent an indolent lymphoma from returning for a longer period of time than after regular doses of chemotherapy. An **allogeneic transplant** (somebody else's bone marrow cells) offers the additional advantage of providing normal stem cells from a healthy donor. Therefore, there is no chance

Allogeneic transplant
a transplant using another individual as the donor.

of lymphoma cells being returned with the transplant. Second, in the case of an allogeneic transplant, an additional and important benefit is the introduction of the donor's immune system. In some types of lymphoma, the donors' immune system can then recognize your lymphoma cells as foreign and destroy them. In this way, an allogeneic transplant is a potential cure for some types of lymphoma. This effect is called **graft versus lymphoma** (GVL). Unfortunately, similar types of immune cells from the healthy donor that cause GVL can cause **graft-versus-host disease** (GVHD). In this condition, the donor's immune cells recognize the patient's body as foreign, attacking certain organs and body parts. GVHD can often be treated and controlled but sometimes can cause a more serious problem or even death. The chance that GVHD will occur and perhaps be more difficult to control rises significantly for older patients. This and other transplant-related problems are reasons why an allogeneic transplant is not often considered a good choice for older patients. GVHD and GVL occur only with an allogeneic transplant. An autologous transplant does not have the benefit of GVL. It therefore relies on the high doses of chemotherapy to cure lymphoma. Because of the immune benefit of GVL, allogeneic transplants do not necessarily need high doses of chemotherapy. Over the past few years, the concept of a **minitransplant** or **nonmyeloablative stem cell transplant** has been introduced as possibly a safer method of performing allogeneic transplants. In this way, the benefit of GVL is becoming increasingly available to older patients who previously would have not been eligible for a regular allogeneic transplant (Table 9 and Question 62).

Graft versus lymphoma

a situation in which the donor's immune system recognizes the recipient's lymphoma cells as foreign and works to eliminate the lymphoma.

Graft-versus-host disease

a situation in which the donor's immune system recognizes the recipient's lymphoma cells as foreign and works to eliminate the lymphoma.

Minitransplant

a transplant in which the doses of chemotherapy or radiotherapy are reduced compared to those given for a standard transplant.

Nonmyeloablative stem cell transplant

same as minitransplant.

Table 9 Different types of bone marrow or blood stem cell transplants

Transplant type	Source of stem cells	Preparative regimen
Autologous	Stem cells obtained from the patient's own blood or bone marrow	High-dose therapy
Allogeneic Sibling Unrelated donor Cord blood transplant	Matched stem cells from a Sibling Volunteer donor Umbilical cord blood stem cell bank	High-dose therapy
Minitransplant (nonmyeloablative)	Sibling or unrelated donor	Reduced-dose therapy

59. What is an autologous transplant?

An autologous transplant uses your own bone marrow or blood stem cells to restore the blood counts after high-dose chemotherapy. The circumstance when an autologous transplant is helpful is one in which the lymphoma is likely to respond to much higher doses of chemotherapy than can be given without the transplant. The higher doses of chemotherapy can also destroy the bone marrow. Therefore, before giving the high-dose therapy, stem cells are collected from the patient and are frozen. After the high-dose chemotherapy, the stem cells are thawed and infused back into the patient. After a period of usually 1.5 to 2 weeks, the stem cells start making all of the different types of blood cells. The cells that recover most rapidly are the white blood cells. The number of stem cells obtained before the transplant affects how fast the stem cells recover. Faster recovery occurs with higher numbers of stem cells. For appropriate patients, the risks of an autologous transplant are low. Because the blood counts drop after the high-dose chemotherapy, there is a higher risk of infection. If this occurs, intravenous antibiotics are required. Platelet transfusions are often needed to reduce the risk of bleeding, and blood transfusions are often required to manage anemia.

Many transplant centers perform autologous transplants on an outpatient basis. When you receive it as an outpatient, it is important that you have someone available at home to help and to drive you to the hospital for the frequent visits (often daily) that are required. If any complication such as a fever occurs, you would be admitted to the hospital.

60. How is an autologous transplant performed?

The procedure for an autologous transplant involves a number of steps. If your lymphoma specialist recommends an autologous transplant, a number of tests are necessary to try to ensure that you are well enough to tolerate the high-dose therapy and the following period of low blood counts. These tests include evaluations of your heart, lung, and kidney function in addition to an assessment of your general well-being. Blood tests to detect any infections, such as hepatitis, will also be obtained. Approval from your insurance company is also required. Next, a **pheresis catheter**, which is usually placed in the upper chest wall, is necessary for collecting stem cells from your blood. **Stem cell mobilization** is the next step, whereby the bone marrow stem cells are stimulated to move into the blood circulation. For stem cell mobilization, white

Pheresis catheter

a large indwelling catheter placed through the skin into a large vein to allow the collection of stem cells.

Stem cell mobilization

the process by which bone marrow stem cells are stimulated to move into blood circulation.

blood cell growth factors given alone or with chemotherapy are administered. The stem cell collection will then be scheduled as the white blood cell count recovers. The collection of the stem cells involves a procedure called **leukapheresis**, for which you are connected to a leukapheresis machine via your pheresis catheter. A small amount of your blood volume is transferred into the machine where the white blood cells are separated from the red blood cells and the platelets. The white cells contain the bone marrow stem cells and are collected in a special bag to be frozen. The red cells and platelets are returned to your circulation. The leukapheresis often needs to be repeated over a few days in order to get an adequate number of stem cells. The procedure on the machine takes approximately 4 to 6 hours.

Leukapheresis
a procedure to remove large numbers of white blood cells from the body.

The stem cells are then frozen along with a chemical protectant which is responsible for the strange garlic-like taste and smell that you may notice when your stem cells are returned to your body. The next stage of the transplant involves managing the side effects of the high-dose chemotherapy and awaiting the recovery of the blood counts. The transplant team will discuss common side effects of the high-dose chemotherapy with you.

61. What are the complications of an autologous transplant?

Problems can relate to having a pheresis catheter, the leukapheresis procedure, the high doses of chemotherapy, and the resulting low blood counts before bone marrow recovery.

Peripheral blood stem cells are collected via a process called apheresis or leukapheresis. This procedure is generally painless, unless you consider boredom to be painful. The leukapheresis machine removes a small amount of your blood volume at a time, separating the bone marrow stem cells from the other blood cells. Patients are closely monitored to ensure that too much blood is not removed at any one time. Sometimes dizziness (lightheadedness or a feeling of faintness) may occur. If so, the machine settings can be adjusted, or a little extra fluid can be given to adjust for the blood volume that is outside of the body at any time. In addition, because the blood outside of the body cannot be allowed to clot, an anticoagulant is added to your blood that can bind calcium. This can result in a fall in the blood calcium that may result in tingling in the fingers and face. Again, adjustments can be made to the machine settings to compensate for these abnormalities, or you may be given extra calcium (such as calcium carbonate [Tums]). Therefore, it is important to inform your nurse if you are experiencing any discomfort. If you have a low platelet count before leukapheresis, the procedure can result in a further fall, and you may need a platelet transfusion before the procedure.

The conditioning or preparative regimens, meaning the high-dose chemotherapy and/or radiation given the week prior to the transplant, vary according to the type of lymphoma being treated, the patient's overall condition, and the medical center in which the transplant is being performed. These treatments may cause nausea and vomiting, which can be prevented with good antinausea drugs; thus, severe nausea is much less common these days. Hair loss, although common, is specific to the combination of drugs used in the conditioning regimen. It usually starts a week or so following the chemotherapy. When this begins, you may prefer to shave your head, as the continuing hair loss can be quite messy. Chemotherapy can damage the lining of the gut. The mouth, all of the way through to the anus, can be affected, resulting in mouth pain, chest pain similar to heartburn, abdominal pain, diarrhea, and rectal pain. Different chemotherapy regimens cause this to varying degrees. Medication can keep you comfortable if the pain becomes unpleasant. A regimen of mouth care that is designed to maintain high levels of oral hygiene will be started with the high-dose chemotherapy. Frequent mouth cleaning with sponges and a mouthwash will lessen the chance of complications, although it may not prevent breakdown. The high doses of chemotherapy can occasionally have damaging effects on other normal body parts. The degree to which this happens depends on the exact type of drug used, and your transplant team will discuss this with you. Possible side effects, which are unusual, include damage to the lungs, heart, liver, bladder, or kidneys. During the time that chemotherapy is given and in the days afterward, you will be examined daily to assess for any evidence of organ damage from the chemotherapy. Blood tests are also obtained for the same reason. Rare complications can arise even after you appear to have completely recovered from the transplant and have returned home. One such side effect relates to the use of a particular nitrosurea alkylating agent used for treating lymphoma and is commonly used in the high-dose therapy regimens. It can cause an inflammation in the lungs, referred to as a pneumonitis, which can result in a cough, a shortness of breath, or a fever developing even up to a year after the transplant. It can be effectively treated with a course of steroids. Therefore, if these symptoms develop, you should contact your physician without delay.

GVHD does not occur after an autologous transplant. Immune-suppressing medications are therefore not required. Patients do not normally need to be on steroids after an autologous transplantation.

Low blood counts are an expected temporary side effect of an autologous transplant, and problems related to it are discussed in Questions 44 and 45.

62. What is an allogeneic transplant?

An allogeneic transplant uses stem cells from a donor. The source of these stem cells can be bone marrow, peripheral blood, or umbilical cord blood. Stem cells are special cells that can produce all three blood cell components. These are white blood cells, red blood cells, and platelets. The donor generally needs to be compatible in terms of genetic similarities. To ensure this, special testing referred to as **human leukocyte antigen (HLA) typing** is performed on both the patient and potential donors.

Human leukocyte antigen typing testing of the transplantation antigens to determine whether two people are compatible for transplantation.

The HLA system consists of a set of different proteins present on most cells in the body. Eight of these proteins are very important for the purposes of a transplant and are transmitted from your parents in two groups of four proteins each. The four proteins in each group are usually passed on together. Each parent provides one set of the proteins to each child. As one of the sets comes from each parent, there is a 25% chance that each brother and sister, as long as they share the same parents, will have the same set of proteins and therefore will have identical HLA. It is rare for other relatives besides brothers or sisters to be HLA identical, as they do not share parents and, therefore, have inherited different HLA proteins. In rare situations, however, it is worthwhile to test children or parents.

If there are no matched siblings, an allogeneic transplant may still be possible, but an unrelated donor would then need to be found. A transplant using an HLA-identical donor other than a sibling is referred to as a matched unrelated donor transplant. An organization, the National Marrow Donor Program, maintains a registry of millions of HLA-typed volunteers who are prepared to donate marrow or peripheral blood stem cells. For HLA typing, a blood sample is obtained, and a bone marrow evaluation is unnecessary. If you are a possible candidate for an unrelated donor transplant, you can be referred to a transplant center, where a search of the registry can be initiated.

The side effects and risks of an allogeneic transplant are quite different from those of an autologous transplant. The fundamental reason is that, along with the new bone marrow cells, you acquire the immune system of your donor. This can be beneficial due to the GVL effect whereby the new immune cells recognize lymphoma cells as foreign and act to eliminate them. This can result in treatment benefits that are unavailable using only chemotherapy. The downside is GVHD (discussed in Question 64).

63. How is an allogeneic transplant performed?

An allogeneic transplant differs from an autologous transplant in a number of ways. Two people are involved—you and your donor. For matched unrelated donor transplants, the National Marrow Donor Program arranges the collection or harvesting of the donor stem cells. These are obtained either directly from the bone marrow during a surgical procedure with general anesthesia or from the blood circulation using leukapheresis. If leukapheresis is performed, as discussed in Question 60, the donor receives a white blood cell growth factor to stimulate stem cells into the blood. Once the stem cells are obtained, they are shipped to the transplant center for infusion into the patient. Before stem cell collection, a physician evaluates and screens the donor for any illness or infectious disease that would make it unsafe. In cases in which the donor is a family member, your transplant physician will arrange for stem cell collection. Once obtained, the stem cells can be either frozen or infused directly into the transplant recipient. Whether they are fresh or frozen, there is no difference in outcome to the recipient. The therapy given to you just before you receive the transplant is designed, except in the case of the minitransplant, to try to eliminate any remaining lymphoma. It is also designed to eliminate your bone marrow and immune system to ensure that your immune system does not reject the new bone marrow cells. The high-dose therapy may consist of chemotherapy alone or may be combined with radiation therapy to the whole body (called total body irradiation). You will generally be hospitalized for these treatments, although in some centers, the radiation may be arranged as an outpatient treatment, usually twice a day over 3 days.

Medications will be provided to prevent nausea and vomiting. After the chemotherapy, a rest day is usual to allow for elimination of drugs from the body. The new bone marrow stem cells are then infused into your bloodstream through a catheter. The day that you receive the new stem cells is referred to as day 0. Then the waiting period for the new cells to start producing all of the blood cells begins. During this period, your blood counts will be low, and the risks for an infection are highest. You will likely also need platelet and red cell transfusions. The chemotherapy or total body irradiation often results in **mucositis**, which can last for a number of days. Morphine may be required for adequate pain control.

Mucositis
inflamation of any of the mucous membranes lining the digestive tract from the mouth, down to the esophogus, to the anus.

Your transplant team will observe you closely to guard against and manage any complications that may arise. After a period of 10 to 14 days, but sometimes as long as 3 weeks, the new stem cells begin to produce blood cells. The white blood count is usually the first of the blood types to recover, often rising to a normal level over a period of only a few days. It is during the time of white cell recovery and the following weeks that graft-versus-host disease is most likely to occur. The platelet count recovers more slowly than the white count.

64. What is graft-versus-host disease?

Graft-versus-host disease (**GVHD**) is the syndrome in which lymphocytes derived from the donor can

GVHD
graft-versus-host-disease

recognize the recipient's body as foreign. The donor lymphocytes essentially attempt to reject the recipient's body. In a kidney or liver transplant patient with a normal immune system, antirejection drugs are given to prevent the patient from rejecting the new kidney or liver. In the case of a bone marrow recipient, his or her immune system has been eliminated, and thus, the new transplanted immune system attempts to reject the recipient. GVHD can be either acute or chronic. Acute GVHD tends to occur when white cells first appear or in the weeks after the transplant. Characteristically, it affects the skin, liver, and/or the gut. It can cause a rash that can affect any area, but in milder cases it may affect only the palms and soles as well as the ear lobes. When the gut is affected, diarrhea occurs. Blood tests or the presence of jaundice detects liver involvement.

GVL
graft-versus-leukemia

Acute GVHD is scored from 1 to 4 according to the severity of the rash, diarrhea, and the abnormal liver tests. If it is grade 1, your transplant physician may choose not to treat it, because some degree of GVHD can be beneficial, as **GVL** may accompany the GVHD. In cases in which the GVHD is more severe, treatment is needed.

The first treatment for GVHD is usually a steroid, which is given orally or intravenously. The medicines used in the attempt to prevent GVHD are also continued. Other medications will be added if the steroids fail to control the GVHD.

Chronic GVHD may occur at any time after the transplant. It may follow directly from acute GVHD or arise without the occurrence of acute GVHD. Chronic GVHD affects individuals differently than does acute GVHD. It may result in dry eyes or a dry mouth. It can affect the skin, resulting in skin thickening. If severe, this can affect the joints, resulting in stiffening.

65. *What are minitransplants?*

The rationale for a minitransplant is discussed in Question 58. Essentially, it is a modification of the traditional allogeneic transplant designed to allow the benefits of GVL to be offered to more patients, including older individuals. The lower dose of chemotherapy or radiation given before receiving the donor stem cells is intended to prevent rejection of the new cells, not to eliminate lymphoma. The idea is that the new immune system will work to eliminate the lymphoma. This takes time, and therefore this type of transplant is not felt to be suitable for patients with rapidly growing lymphoma. Also, the best GVL effect is seen among patients with indolent lymphoma. It appears likely that the complication rate for this sort of transplant is lower, partly because it has less effect on normal body tissues from the lower doses of chemotherapy. Tissue damage contributes to GVHD by releasing cytokines. In the minitransplant setting, this is minimized with—it is hoped—less GVHD while still allowing GVL to occur. One major research goal in transplant is to separate the cells causing GVHD from those that can cause GVL. Currently, this goal remains elusive.

66. When should I have a transplant?

This is a complicated issue and depends on your type of lymphoma, your response to previous treatment, your age, and your overall general condition. The answer is therefore addressed depending on lymphoma type.

Indolent Lymphoma

Because indolent lymphoma tends to occur in older individuals, most patients are not candidates for an allogeneic transplant. A minitransplant can be considered in certain circumstances. An HLA-matching sibling is usually required, but often a matched unrelated donor is also accepted. Some studies suggest that this type of transplant may actually cure some patients. The possibility of a cure results from the GVL effect. This treatment option should be considered, especially in younger patients with a suitable donor.

An autologous transplant is an option for a greater number of patients. It does not provide a cure, but in many instances it can provide an extended period before the lymphoma returns. Extending the time before another course of treatment is needed may be a significant advantage for many patients.

Purging
the technique whereby certain cells (usually cancerous) are removed from the remaining cells present in the collected bone marrow or stem cells.

Many clinical studies are being conducted in an attempt to improve the results of autologous transplants. Such studies include attempts to purge the bone marrow stem cells before the transplant. **Purging** refers to the removal of any lymphoma cells that may contaminate the stem cells. Methods of purging include treating the stem cells in the laboratory with chemotherapy or antibodies targeting lymphoma cells. This is called ex vivo purging. Treating the patient with chemotherapy or antibodies before collecting the stem cells is a method of in vivo purging. It is not yet clear whether purging results in a better outcome. Ongoing studies are addressing prevention of lymphoma recurrence after an autologous transplant. Such approaches include the use of maintenance therapy with monoclonal antibody treatments or vaccination strategies.

Aggressive Lymphoma

The aggressive lymphomas include the intermediate- and high-grade lymphomas. The GVL effect that can cure some indolent lymphomas appears to be less effective for these lymphomas. Therefore, an allogeneic transplant is performed less frequently for these disorders. However, for many patients whose lymphoma returns after the initial chemotherapy an autologous transplant is often the next recommended treatment (Question 59). Remember, these lymphomas can still be cured with a transplant. As previously noted, patients whose lymphoma continues to respond to regular doses of chemotherapy are the best candidates for transplantation. There may also be patients who, at the time their lymphoma is first diagnosed, appear to be at a particularly high risk of the lymphoma recurring after chemotherapy. The IPI can help to identify such patients. Currently, clinical studies are ongoing, attempting to determine whether performing an autologous transplant immediately after completing the first course of chemotherapy can prevent the lymphoma from recurring, thereby increasing the cure rate.

67. Should I seek complementary therapy?

Conventional therapies, including such treatments as chemotherapy, monoclonal antibody therapy, and radiation therapy, are treatments that medical doctors recommend. These treatments have been demonstrated in clinical trials to provide the most anticancer activity. Obviously, these treatments are far from perfect, and much work remains to be done. Because of the failings of conventional treatments, interest in **complementary therapy** and alternative therapy is high.

Complementary therapy
therapy used in conjunction with traditional medical treatments.

Complementary therapies are techniques or approaches that are used in addition to standard or conventional treatments. Examples include meditation, acupuncture, relaxation and massage, visualization, and diet and herbal regimens. Many of these treatments are derived from traditional healing practices and can be important additions to the more traditional treatments. They often help individuals to cope better and feel more in control. Oncologists recognize many complementary therapies for their positive effects on a patient's sense of well-being. The medical community accepts and encourages therapies such as relaxation and visualization. In many cancer centers, you can receive instruction and learn the techniques of various complementary therapies. It is advisable to discuss these therapies with your physician. Rarely, there may be specific reasons why you should avoid a specific complementary therapy.

Meditation and relaxation have been demonstrated to help obtain relief from nausea, anxiety, depression, and stress. Many ways exist to practice meditation and relaxation, and many books and tapes are available at libraries and bookstores. You may need to experiment with a few different techniques before you find one that works for you.

The positive effects of such complementary techniques on the outcome of lymphoma are unknown. Although there is no concrete evidence that such techniques can directly influence lymphoma, indirect effects may exist via subtle changes in the immune system. No harm is brought from such interventions, especially if they help patients to feel more in control. Additional information can be obtained from the National Center for Complementary and Alternative Medicine. Its website is at www.nccam.nih.gov.

68. Should I seek alternative therapy?

Alternative therapy, in contrast to complementary therapy, is the substitution of standard medical treatments with unproven and unconventional treatments. In many cases, even lymphoma that has recurred may be curable, so it is heartbreaking to see vulnerable patients decline such potentially curable therapy for alternative remedies without proven benefit. The use of such therapies may result in the loss of an opportunity for a cure.

Alternative therapy
a therapy other than a conventionally accepted medical treatment.

Lymphoma patients, like all cancer patients, are vulnerable and may be disillusioned with their physician or medical clinic or feel bitter as a result of a relapse. In these situations, it is natural to reach out toward any hope.

Many claims are made for many different remedies. Often, the actual nature of the remedy is not disclosed, and such treatments may cost large sums of money. Usually little or no evidence supports the use of the remedy apart from a list of testimonials from cured patients.

We would simply advise caution. You expect your lymphoma specialist to have a good rationale for the treatments that he or she prescribes. Hold alternative therapy practitioners to the same standard. Often, alternative therapy practitioners will state that only large pharmaceutical companies can afford to conduct such research. It has been suggested that these same companies even obstruct alternative therapy practitioners from conducting such research. Whatever the reason for the lack of studies and evidence regarding these treatments, it is unconscionable to make such exaggerated claims about expensive products to vulnerable patients. Furthermore, patients are often led to believe that the failure of a product was due to their lack of effort or belief in the product, and that with only more effort or belief (and of course expense) benefit may arise.

69. What are clinical trials?

Clinical trials are the mechanism by which new and safer treatments are evaluated. They aim to determine whether a treatment is effective, whether it is better than existing treatments, and whether the treatment can be administered safely. It is only through carefully performed clinical trials that potential new treatments can be transferred from the laboratory to the bedside.

In the development of a new drug, preclinical studies are the first step. These are studies performed in laboratories and/or animals (usually mice) that provide the first indication that the drug has some activity directed against a cancer. If a drug appears promising, a phase 1 study may be performed, which is primarily conducted to determine the correct dose of the new treatment and to obtain further information about side effects. Most phase 1 studies are designed to start off at a very low dose of the medication in small groups of patients. The patients are monitored closely for the development of any side effects. If no side effects are seen, another small group of patients will be treated at a higher dose. In this fashion, subsequent patients receive increasing doses of the drug, assuming that the patients treated at the lower dose levels tolerated the medication without unacceptable side effects. In this way, the effect of the drug in humans can be assessed in a relatively safe manner. Of course, there are risks to participating in a phase 1 trial. Although unexpected side effects may exist, the possibility of obtaining a significant benefit also has potential. Often, it is patients whose cancer is progressing in spite of previous treatments who are most willing to participate in phase 1 clinical trials.

After completing phase 1, new treatments enter phase 2 studies. Once the correct dose and side effects are known, the phase 2 study is to establish that a treatment is effective. A phase 2 study involves a larger group of patients who all generally receive the same dose. They are evaluated to determine how the cancer responds to the treatment and also to gather further information about side effects.

If the treatment still appears promising, it will continue into phase 3, which is usually designed to compare the new treatment with other currently available treatments. This phase often involves a randomized study in which patients have a 1 in 2 chance of receiving the new treatment. Patients are then followed closely, and the response of patients in the two groups is compared. It is preferable that neither the patient nor his or her physician is aware of which treatment is administered, as this could lead to bias in favor of one treatment over another. A phase 3 study is the best method for demonstrating that one treatment is better than another. The Food and Drug Administration has a mandate to regulate medications. Before approval for use, all clinical trial data are reviewed to ensure that a drug meets the standards for being safe and effective.

Only through clinical trials can patients and their doctors know which treatments are best for their type of cancer. A new treatment gets evaluated because there are indications that it may be more effective, safer, or easier on the patient than an alternative treatment. Drugs that do not show promise are not further evaluated. If clinical trials were not conducted, physicians would have nothing concrete to guide them when making recommendations to patients. Treatments currently used for lymphoma are the direct result of previous patients volunteering for clinical trials.

Patients entering a clinical trial are not guinea pigs. Before a clinical trial can enroll patients, it is carefully reviewed from scientific, safety, and ethical viewpoints. Patients also need to provide informed consent, which establishes that they understand the reason for the study, the risks and possible benefits, and the availability of alternative treatment options. **Institutional review boards** are required to approve and monitor the conduct of clinical trials and have the ability to suspend or close a trial if there are concerns about safety.

Institutional review board

(commonly termed the IRB) a group that reviews research studies to ensure they are safe and ethical.

A drug company with an interest in developing a particular drug may sponsor a clinical trial, or the funding may come from an independent source such as a university grant or a government agency. The same strict requirements need to be followed regardless of the source of funding.

70. Should I enter a clinical trial?

Participation in a clinical trial can be beneficial in many respects. You may be eligible to participate in various trials depending on your type and grade of lymphoma. Your overall condition and the treatment you have already received are also factors to be considered. Discuss with your lymphoma doctor whether any suitable clinical trials are available, as they often offer a way for receiving new and innovative treatments that otherwise may be unavailable. Patients in a clinical trial also receive very close medical supervision and monitoring.

Participation in a clinical trial can be beneficial in many respects. You may be eligible to participate in various trials depending on your type and grade of lymphoma.

Clinical trials are necessary because they help expand the knowledge base of lymphoma and the best treatment options now and in the future. Participants of clinical trials may have the opportunity to benefit from treatments that have shown promise in earlier research.

Cancer centers often have a number of clinical trials available for different cancers. Smaller oncology practices, however, may have few or no trials available. Participation in a trial may then require travel away from home and loved ones. Because a clinical trial cannot offer any guarantee of benefit, the disruption and inconvenience may outweigh the benefit and can also be a significant emotional and financial burden for you and your family.

When deciding on participation in a clinical trial, collect as much information as possible. Find out what the treatment involves, how it is different from standard treatments, and what the relative risks and benefits are. Ask whether any other clinical trials are available and what the experience has been to date. Inquire whether the trial is phase 1, phase 2, or phase 3, and ask what question the trial is hoping to answer.

Before making a final decision, ensure that you have a very good understanding of the treatment involved and also of the time commitment. Find out whether there are any costs for which you are responsible. Also, try to develop an understanding of the likelihood of benefit from the treatment. Often, participating in a clinical trial is the right decision, especially at times when few other options are available, patients are vulnerable to and may reach out toward anything offering a glimmer of hope. Thoughtful discussion with your physician and sometimes a second opinion may help you to make a rational decision.

71. How do I find out what clinical trials are available?

Most patients receive information about treatment options from their lymphoma physician. However, you can also find out about clinical trials from the National Cancer Institute. Someone at the institute can be contacted at 1-800-422-6237 or on its website at www.clinicaltrials.gov. Other websites with helpful information are included in the Appendix.

PART SIX

Coping with Lymphoma

Can I continue to work?

Should I join a support group?

If I am dying, how do I cope?

More . . .

72. Can I continue to work?

The ability of someone to continue working after their diagnosis of lymphoma depends on several factors. These include the type of work involved, the schedule and time demands of the treatment, and the side effects of the treatment. There are people who feel very well and have little or no side effects from their treatment, and their overall strength and endurance are not affected. They have their treatment first thing in the morning and are able to go directly to work. Many people feel that work is a fundamental part of their life. Continuing to work can provide a sense of structure, stability, and normalcy. It is also an opportunity for you to interact with your peers. Even if you are able to continue to work, it's a good idea to discuss your diagnosis with your employer, because you will need to take time off for medical appointments and treatments. Your employer will be much more understanding if he or she is aware of the reasons for your absence.

Many people, however, feel impaired and may require rest during the day. If you decide to not work, it's a good idea to contact your employer's human resources department, as they can inform you of the steps necessary to ensure that your medical insurance is not interrupted. You may also benefit from talking to a social worker about your eligibility for disability benefits.

73. Should I join a support group?

Support groups, which are available in most communities, may be designed for all cancer patients or for only lymphoma patients. Support groups usually meet monthly, and family members are generally welcome to attend. A support group may also be available specifically for family members.

Your attendance in a support group does not necessarily require that you open up to the group, because you may simply prefer to listen. Often it is comforting to hear the stories of how others cope with a similar illness, and you may gain some very helpful insights. If you are unsure whether you will benefit from attendance, try it once or twice, as there is no obligation to continue. Remember, however, that you may also be able to provide much comfort, support, inspiration, and advice to others in the group, especially if you continue to do well. For contact information, ask your physician, nurse, or social worker. The American Cancer Society and the Leukemia and Lymphoma Society have chapter offices throughout the United States.

74. If I am dying, how do I cope?

Because coming to terms with one's death is very difficult for most of us, advanced preparations can help. Honesty and openness with loved ones and friends are very important. Honest communication between the medical team and the patient is also very important. Death is a difficult subject for most of us to discuss, and this is certainly true of most physicians, even oncology and hematology physicians. Too frequently, this subject will not be adequately discussed, sometimes resulting in a sense of mistrust and suspicion between patients and their family members and physicians. It is very important that up-front discussions be held regarding the appropriateness of further treatment when it is unlikely to provide benefit. Patients

Accepting that further treatment is futile can actually be a very empowering time. It can remove much stress and allow you to dedicate your remaining time to those who are most important to you.

may wish to continue treatment, even with little hope of any meaningful response. Having the ability to accept that further treatment is unlikely to be beneficial and may actually be harmful is a great step forward in accepting death. Trust in your physician is essential in reaching this realization. Even if further treatment is not physically harmful, it can deprive you of meaningful quality of life. Accepting that further treatment is futile can actually be a very empowering time. It can remove much stress and allow you to dedicate your remaining time to those who are most important to you. You may feel physically much better, as further side effects of treatment are avoided. Talking to a minister or social worker can also be helpful.

Once the decision is made not to pursue further active treatment against the lymphoma, hospice may be appropriate. The hospice movement, in which the emphasis is on quality of life and symptom and pain management, rather than the length of life, has evolved greatly over the past 100 years. Most hospice facilities provide support to patients in their own home as much as possible.

Durable power of attorney

a document allowing another person, usually a close relative, to make financial and medical decisions in the event that you are incapacitated.

Advance directive

a legal document that clarifies a patient's wishes in advance in the event he is unable to make decisions at a later time and allows the assignment of an alternative individual to make such decisions.

Advance planning for serious illness includes an advance directive and a **durable power of attorney**. An **advance directive** is a document that states your preferences for treatments that you will or will not accept if you are in a position in which you are unable to make such a decision. This may be the only way the medical team knows and can honor your wishes. Advance directive forms are available from your healthcare facility. An advance directive may cover such issues as a **"do not resuscitate" order**, which addresses your wishes concerning resuscitation in the event of heart or lung failure. Because resuscitation usually involves life-support apparatus, your decision about this should be made in advance.

A durable power of attorney or a healthcare proxy allows a specific family member to make decisions about your health care in the event that you are incapacitated. The durable power of attorney also allows an individual to make financial and legal decisions.

Do not resuscitate order
a state whereby aggressive life-saving measures, such as cardiopulmonary resuscitation (CPR), will not be undertaken because they are unlikely to prolong useful life.

75. What happens if I have no insurance or insufficient insurance coverage?

Patients without insurance (and sometimes even for those with insurance) must carry a significant financial burden because of their illness. The hospital or clinic will tell you to whom you should speak regarding financial options. Most healthcare facilities will have a financial caseworker or social worker to direct you toward some help. Government programs, disability benefits, or volunteer organizations may provide helpful resources.

The American Cancer Society has a list of useful resources on its website (www.cancer.org), which includes information regarding Medicaid and Medicare eligibility, and makes the following recommendations regarding dealings with your insurance company:

- Become familiar with your individual insurance plan and its provisions. If you think that you might need additional insurance, ask your insurance carrier whether it is available.
- Submit claims for all medical expenses even when you are uncertain about your coverage.

- Keep accurate and complete records of claims submitted, pending, and paid.
- Keep copies of all paperwork related to your claims, such as letters of medical necessity, bills, receipts, requests for sick leave, and correspondence with insurance companies.
- Get a caseworker, a hospital financial counselor, or a social worker to help you if your finances are limited. Often, companies or hospitals can work with you to make acceptable payment arrangements if you make them aware of your situation.
- Submit your bills as you receive them. If you become overwhelmed with bills, get help. Contact local support organizations, such as your American Cancer Society or your state's government agencies, for additional assistance.
- Do not allow your medical insurance to expire. Pay premiums in full and on time, as it is often very difficult to get new insurance.

Organizations

The American Cancer Society
American Cancer Society National Home Office
1599 Clifton Road
Atlanta, GA 30329
Phone: 800-ACS-2345
Website: www.cancer.org

American Society of Clinical Oncology
1900 Duke Street, Suite 200
Alexandria, VA 22314
Phone: 703-299-0150
Fax: 703-299-1044
Website: www.asco.org

American Society of Hematology
1900 M Street NW, Suite 200
Washington, DC 20036
Phone: 202-776-0544
Fax: 202-776-0545
Website: www.hematology.org

Blood and Marrow Transplant Information Network
2900 Skokie Valley Road, Suite B
Highland Park, IL 60035
Phone: 888-597-7674 or 847-433-3313
Website: www.bmtinfonet.org

The Bone Marrow Foundation
70 East 55th Street, 20th Floor
New York, NY 10022
Phone: 800-365-1336
Website: www.bonemarrow.org

Cancer Care, Inc.
275 7th Avenue
New York, NY 10001
Phone: 212-712-8400 (administration); 212-712-8080 (services)
Website: www.cancercare.org

Cancer Research Institute
681 Fifth Avenue
New York, NY 10022
Phone: 800-99-CANCER (800-992-2623)
Website: www.cancerresearch.org

The Center for International Bone and Marrow Transplant Research
Froedtert and the Medical College of Wisconsin Clinical Cancer Center
9200 W. Wisconsin Ave
Suite C5500
Milwaukee, WI 53226
Phone: 414-805-0700
Website: www.cibmtr.org

Cure for Lymphoma Foundation
215 Lexington Ave, 11th Floor
New York, NY 10016
Phone: 800-235-6848 or 212-213-9595
Website: www.lymphoma.org

Department of Veterans Affairs
Veterans Health Association
810 Vermont Avenue, NW
Washington, DC 20420
Phone: 202-273-5400 (Washington, DC office)
800-827-1000 (local VA office)
Website: www.va.gov

Leukemia & Lymphoma Society of America
Phone: 800-955-4572 for local chapter information
Website: www.leukemia-lymphoma.org

Lymphoma Research Foundation
111 Broadway, 19th Floor
New York, NY 10006
Phone: 212-349-2910 or 800-235-6848
or
8800 Venice Boulevard, Suite 207
Los Angeles, CA 90034
Phone: 310-204-7040 or 800-500-9976
Website: www.lymphoma.org

National Cancer Institute
National Cancer Institute Public Information Office
Building 31, Room 10A31
31 Center Drive, MSC 2580
Bethesda, MD 20892-2580
Phone: 301-435-3848 (public information office line)
Website: www.nci.nih.gov
For clinical trial information: www.clinicaltrials.gov

National Center for Complementary and Alternative Medicine
NCCAM Clearinghouse
PO Box 7923
Gaithersburg, MD 20898
Phone: 888-644-6226
Website: www.nccam.nih.gov

National Coalition for Cancer Survivorship
1010 Wayne Avenue, Suite 770
Silver Spring, MD 20910
Phone: 301-650-9127
Website: www.canceradvocacy.org

National Comprehensive Cancer Network
50 Huntingdon Pike, Suite 200
Rockledge, PA 19046
Phone: 888-909-NCCN (888-909-6226)
Website: www.nccn.org

National Marrow Donor Program (NMDP)
3001 Broadway St NE, Suite 500
Minneapolis, MN 55413
Phone: 800-654-1247 or 612-627-5800
Website: www.marrow.org

Office of Patient Advocacy
Phone: 888-999-6743
Website: www.marrow.org

Oncology Nursing Society
501 Holiday Drive
Pittsburgh, PA 15220
Phone: 412-921-7373
Website: www.ons.org

Social Security Administration
Office of Public Inquiries
6401 Security Boulevard, Room 4-C–5 Annex
Baltimore, MD 21235-6401
Phone: 800-772-1213 or 800-325-0778 (TTY)
Website: www.ssa.gov

United Seniors Health Cooperative (USHC)
USHC, Suite 200
409 Third Street, SW
Washington, DC 20024
Phone: 800-637-2604 or 202-479-6973
Website: www.unitedseniorshealth.org

The Wellness Community
8044 Montgomery Road, Suite 170
Cincinnati, OH 45236
Phone: 888-793-WELL (888-793-9355)
Website: www.cancer-support.org

Well Spouse Foundation
30 E. 40th Street
New York, NY 10016
Phone: 800-838-0879 or 212-685-8815
Website: www.wellspouse.org

Additional Websites with Lymphoma Information

Association of Cancer Online Resources
www.acor.org

Cancer.Net
www.cancer.net

Lymphoma Information Network
www.lymphomainfo.net

Other Websites of Interest

www.aicr.org
The American Institute for Cancer Research
This site discusses methods to reduce the risk of cancer.

www.cancersupportivecare.com/pharmacy.html
This site covers chemotherapy drugs and ways of coping with their side effects. It also has links to the financial assistance programs of pharmaceutical companies.

www.cms.hhs.gov
This is the website for the Centers for Medicare and Medicaid Services.

www.dol.gov
Information on the Family and Medical Leave Act can be found here.

www.needymeds.com
This is an information site for patient financial assistance programs for medications.

www.usda.gov/cnpp/
The U.S. Department of Agriculture; Center for Nutrition Policy and Promotion. This website focuses on healthy eating habits.

Glossary

Acquired immunodeficiency syndrome (AIDS): the syndrome resulting from infection with the human immunodeficiency virus (HIV).

Advance directive: a legal document that clarifies a patient's wishes in advance in the event he is unable to make decisions at a later time and allows the assignment of an alternative individual to make such decisions.

Alkylating agents: a class of chemotherapy drugs.

Allogeneic transplant: a transplant using another individual as the donor.

Alopecia: hair loss.

Alternative therapy: a therapy other than a conventionally accepted medical treatment.

Anemia: a low hemoglobin level.

Anemia of chronic disease: an anemia caused by the bone marrow's reaction to being sick.

Ann Arbor Staging System: used to describe the areas in the body affected by the lymphoma. It was created at a conference held in Ann Arbor, Michigan.

Anorexia: loss of appetite.

Antibodies: specialized proteins of the immune system that help fight infections. They can also be created to recognize proteins on cancer cells, as in some types of lymphoma treatments.

Antibody therapy: the use of antibodies to treat cancer.

Anti-CD20 monoclonal antibody: A class of drugs that inactivates the molecule called CD20, present on the surface of B-cells (which can become cancerous).

Antiemetic: a medication to prevent nausea and vomiting.

Antigen: any substance that can induce an immune response. This could be an infection or a cancer cell.

Antitumor antibiotics: a class of chemotherapy drugs.

Aorta: the main blood vessel (artery) that carries blood from the heart to the smaller arteries, delivering blood to all parts of the body.

Aplasia: a condition where blood cells are not produced.

Apoptosis: a process by which normal cells die. Some cancer cells do not die, and a failure of cells to undergo apoptosis can contribute to the growth of cancer. It is often referred to as "programmed cell death."

Arteries: the vessels that carry blood containing oxygen to the organs and tissues of the body.

Autoimmune disease: an illness in which the person's own immune system can recognize parts of its own body as foreign.

Autologous stem cell transplant: a transplant in which one is one's own bone marrow stem cell donor.

B cells: a type of lymphocyte.

B symptoms: fevers, night sweats, and weight loss that may occur in lymphoma patients. They can occur individually or together.

Bacteria: one class of infectious agents.

Basophils: a type of white blood cell.

Benign: not cancerous.

Biologic therapy: treatment that focuses the body's immune system on diseased cells.

Biopsy: the removal of tissue or a fluid sample for microscopic examination.

Bolus: a rapid intravenous injection.

Bone marrow: soft substance inside many bones in the body where the blood cells are produced.

Broviac catheter: a type of catheter that goes directly into a large vein to allow easier administration of medications and blood tests.

CD20: a protein on the surface of B lymphocytes and most B cell lymphomas.

Cellular immune response: the part of the immune response that uses lymphocytes to directly remove antigens. In contrast, the humoral immune response uses antibodies to remove antigens.

Central nervous system: the brain and spinal cord.

Chemotherapy: drugs used to treat a disease; the different types of drugs used to treat cancer.

Chronic lymphocytic leukemia: the most common slow-growing type of leukemia.

Clinical trials: research studies evaluating promising new treatments in patients.

Complementary therapy: therapies used in conjunction with traditional medical treatments.

Complete blood count: a blood test looking at the red blood cell count, the hemoglobin, the white blood cell count, and the platelet count.

Computed tomography (CT) scan: a specialized type of X-ray that creates a detailed cross-sectional view of the body.

Contrast dye: a chemical that is injected for certain X-rays, including CT scans and MRI scans, that results in better contrast pictures.

Cytokines: chemicals produced by T lymphocytes to generate an immune response.

Cytoplasm: the part of a cell that surrounds the central nucleus.

Dehydration: low fluids in the body, which can cause dizziness, fatigue, fainting, and other minor symptoms. If not corrected, dehydration can cause more serious problems.

Deoxyribonucleic acid (DNA): the material that carries the genetic code for each organism or person.

Depression: a disorder characterized by excessive sadness and feelings of hopelessness.

Diaphragm: the large muscle that separates the lungs from the abdomen. Its movement is important for breathing.

Diffuse large B cell lymphoma: a type of intermediate-grade lymphoma.

Dimples of Venus: the dimples seen on the skin over the sacrum on the lower back.

Do not resuscitate order: a state whereby aggressive life-saving measures, such as cardiopulmonary resuscitation (CPR), will not be undertaken because they are unlikely to prolong useful life.

Durable power of attorney: a document allowing another person, usually a close relative, to make financial and medical decisions in the event that one is incapacitated.

Enzymes: chemical messengers within the body.

Eosinophil: a type of white blood cell.

Epstein-Barr virus: the virus that causes infectious mononucleosis and can cause lymphocytes to grow abnormally.

Erythropoietin: a hormone produced by the kidneys that stimulates the bone marrow to produce red blood cells.

Esophagitis: inflammation of the esophagus.

Esophagus: the tube connecting the throat to the stomach.

Fatigue: tiredness, particularly the debilitating, continuous tiredness that signals illness or disease.

Femur: the thigh bone.

Fine needle aspiration (FNA): a procedure to obtain a sample of tissue using a small needle.

Flow cytometry: a procedure for examining the proteins present on the surface of cells.

Follicles: round structures containing lymphocytes.

Follicular lymphomas: lymphomas composed of lymphocytes organized into round structures.

Follicular Lymphoma International Prognostic Index (FLIPI): a modified form of the IPI for determining the prognosis of patients with follicular lymphomas.

Gallium scan: a nuclear medicine test that uses gallium to show areas of lymphoma within the body.

Gamma camera: a nuclear imaging camera that can detect radioactivity.

Gastrointestinal tract: the gut, from mouth to anus.

Graft-versus-host disease: an illness caused by the donor's immune system recognizing and attacking tissues and organs of the marrow recipient.

Graft-versus-lymphoma: a situation in which the donor's immune system recognizes the recipient's lymphoma cells as foreign and works to eliminate the lymphoma.

Granules: small particles containing enzymes.

Growth factors: chemicals that can be injected to stimulate the production of blood cells.

Hematocrit: a measure of the number of red cells, useful for anemia or polycythemia (too many red cells).

Hematologist/oncologist: a physician specializing in the treatment of blood disorders and cancer.

Hematology: the study of diseases of the blood, including blood cancers.

Hematopoietic stem cell: the most immature cell that develops into red blood cells, white blood cells, and platelets.

Hemoglobin: a protein present in red blood cells that carries oxygen.

Hepatitis C virus: one of the viruses that can infect the liver and cause chronic liver inflammation.

Hickman catheter: an intravenous line that passes through the skin into a large vein near the heart. It provides a safer and easier way to administer chemotherapy and obtain blood samples.

Human immunodeficiency virus (HIV): a virus that attacks the human immune system, leaving the carrier prone to infections.

Human leukocyte antigen typing: testing of the transplantation antigens to determine whether two people are compatible for transplantation.

Humerus: the major bone connecting the shoulder to the elbow.

Humoral immune response: an immune response that uses antibodies rather than cells to destroy an antigen (foreign protein).

Idiotype: a protein sequence on the surface of B lymphocytes that is like a fingerprint. All related lymphocytes contain the same protein sequence.

Immune system: the complex system by which the body protects itself from harmful outside invaders.

Immunotherapy: treatment aimed at controlling the immune system.

Indolent: usually slow growing.

Indwelling catheter: an intravenous catheter that can remain in place for longer than a few days.

Infectious mononucleosis: a viral infection caused by the Epstein-Barr virus. Also called glandular fever.

Inferior vena cava: the large vein that carries blood back toward the heart.

Institutional review board: (commonly termed the IRB) a group that reviews research studies to ensure they are safe and ethical.

International Prognostic Index (IPI): a system to determine the prognosis of patients with lymphoma.

Interventional radiologist: a physician who is trained in using X-rays to aid in the performance of some types of surgical procedures.

Intramuscular: an injection into the muscle.

Intrathecal: an injection into the fluid surrounding the spinal cord or brain.

Karnofsky Performance Status scale: a system to evaluate how patients do when performing normal daily activities.

Lactate dehydrogenase: an enzyme measured using a simple blood test.

Laparotomy: surgery involving an incision to look directly into the abdomen.

Leukapheresis: a procedure to remove large numbers of white blood cells from the body.

Leukopenia: a low white blood cell count.

Libido: sex drive.

Local treatment: treatment aimed at a particular area of the body. For example, radiation treatment is local, whereas chemotherapy is systemic.

Low microbial diet: a diet containing low amounts of bacteria or fungi.

Lymph fluid: the fluid that carries lymphocytes around the body.

Lymph glands: the large collections of lymphocytes present at intervals throughout the lymph system. They can get big and painful in response to an infection.

Lymph node architecture: the structure of lymph nodes when they are seen under a microscope.

Lymph nodes: another term for lymph glands.

Lymphadenopathy: enlarged lymph nodes.

Lymphangiogram: an X-ray study of lymph glands after they are injected with a dye.

Lymphatic channels: the tiny vessels that connect the lymph glands.

Lymphocytes: the main type of cell that makes up the immune system and is the abnormal cell in lymphoma.

Lymphokines: chemicals that are produced by lymphocytes and help in coordinating the immune response.

Lymphoma: cancer of the lymphocytes.

Lymphoma classification: a system to organize the many different types of lymphoma.

Magnetic resonance imaging: a technique based on the use of magnetic fields to produce images of body parts.

Malaria: an infection caused by a parasite and transmitted by mosquitoes.

Malignant: cancerous.

Mediastinal nodes: lymph nodes present in the area between the lungs.

Megakaryocytes: the bone marrow cells that produce platelets.

Megestrol acetate: a medication that can increase the appetite.

Mesenteric lymph nodes: the lymph nodes present in the abdomen tissue that anchors the bowel.

Microtubules: structures present in individual cells that are important for allowing cells to divide.

Minitransplant: a transplant in which the doses of chemotherapy or radiotherapy are reduced compared to those given for a standard transplant.

Monoclonal antibodies: antibodies that bind to a specific target on the surface of lymphoma or other cancer cells.

Monocyte: a type of white blood cell.

Mucositis: Inflammation of any of the mucous membranes lining the digestive tract from the mouth, down to the esophagus, to the anus.

Neutropenia: a low level of neutrophils

Neutrophil: the main white blood cell important for fighting infection.

Nodules: see Follicles.

Non-Hodgkin's lymphoma: the most common type of lymphoma.

Nonmyeloablative stem cell transplant: see minitransplant.

Nuclear medicine: the medicine specialty that deals with using radioisotopes for obtaining body scans and for treatment.

Nucleoside analogue: a type of chemotherapy drug that targets lymphocytes.

Nucleus: the central part of the cell that contains the genetic information.

Oncology: the field of medicine that studies cancer.

Palpitations: the sensation of an irregular heartbeat.

Pathologist: a physician who makes the diagnosis of lymphoma and other cancers from evaluating biopsies and other surgical specimens under the microscope.

Performance status: the level of ability with which patients can perform their routine daily activities.

Peripheral blood stem cell transplant: a transplant using marrow stem cells that have been obtained from the blood circulation.

PET scan: see Positron emission tomography.

Petechiae: pinpoint red spots that occur with low platelet counts and are due to tiny areas of bleeding into the skin.

Phagocyte: a cell that scavenges other cells.

Pheresis catheter: a large indwelling catheter placed through the skin into a large vein to allow the collection of stem cells.

Plasma cells: the most mature type of B cell. They produce immunoglobulins.

Platelets: the tiny blood cells that are produced in the bone marrow and are important for blood clotting.

Pneumocystis carinii pneumoniae: an infection affecting the lungs that can occur in people with an abnormal immune system.

Portacath: an indwelling intravenous catheter that is placed entirely underneath the skin.

Positron emission tomography (PET): X-ray studies that use the abnormal sugar metabolism of cancer cells to identify metastatic deposits.

Power of attorney: see Durable power of attorney.

Prognosis: a prediction of the course that a disease will take.

Pulmonary function tests: a set of tests performed to evaluate the ability of the lungs to function properly.

Purging: the technique whereby certain cells (usually cancerous) are removed from the remaining cells present in the collected bone marrow or stem cells.

Radiation therapy: treatment using radiation.

Red blood cells: the most common type of blood cells that carry oxygen around the body.

Reproductive system: the body parts associated with reproduction.

Retroperitoneal lymph nodes: the most common lymph nodes present in the abdomen.

Revised European-American Classification: the basis of the newest lymphoma classification.

Rheumatoid arthritis: an autoimmune disorder associated with destruction and deformity of joints.

Saliva: the lubricating substance produced by the salivary glands that is essential for chewing and swallowing.

Shingles: a painful condition with a rash, usually affecting one area of the skin in the distribution of a nerve. It is due to reactivation of the chickenpox virus and usually occurs when the immune system is depressed.

Simulation: the planning necessary before administering any radiation treatment.

Small lymphocytic lymphoma: a type of indolent lymphoma that is similar to chronic lymphocytic leukemia.

Spinal fluid: the fluid surrounding the brain and spinal fluid.

Spinal tap: the procedure for obtaining a sample of spinal fluid.

Spleen: the large lymph node–like organ under the lower left ribs.

Stage: a reference to the number of places in the body affected by lymphoma or other cancer.

Stem cell mobilization: the process by which bone marrow stem cells are stimulated to move into blood circulation.

Stem cells: the cells that can produce red blood cells, white blood cells, and platelets.

Subcutaneous: underneath the skin.

Superior vena cava syndrome: a condition in which the blood flow back to the heart is decreased due to obstruction, usually by very big lymph nodes.

Systemic lupus erythematosus: a disease in which the immune system attacks the body.

Systemic treatment: a treatment, such as chemotherapy, that reaches all body parts through the bloodstream.

T cells: one of the major types of lymphocytes.

Testosterone: a male hormone.

Thrombocytopenia: a low platelet count.

Thymus: an organ behind the breastbone that is important for the development of an immune response, especially in children.

Tissues: a collection of cells of a similar type with a similar function.

Tonsils: large lymph nodes present in the back of the throat.

Total body irradiation: radiation therapy administered to the entire body, usually in preparation for a transplant.

Translocation: an abnormality of certain chromosomes seen in some cancer cells.

Vaccine: a preparation of a protein given to stimulate an immune response against a particular infection.

Veins: blood vessels that return blood to the heart.

Vinca alkaloids: a type of chemotherapy drug.

Viruses: tiny infectious agents that require other cells for their growth and survival.

White blood cells: blood cells that are most important for fighting infection.

Working Formulation: one of the lymphoma classifications.

Xerostomia: dryness of the mouth due to disease.

Index

page numbers followed by *f* denote figures, *t* denote tables

A

D

E

F

G

M

N